Diagnosis of Endometriosis

Diagnosis of Endometriosis: Biomarkers and Clinical Methods

Editor

Antonio Simone Laganà

MDPI • Basel • Beijing • Wuhan • Barcelona • Belgrade • Manchester • Tokyo • Cluj • Tianjin

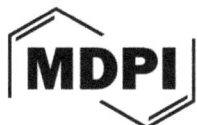

Editor
Antonio Simone Laganà
Department of Obstetrics and
Gynecology
"Filippo Del Ponte" Hospital
University of Insubria
Varese
Italy

Editorial Office
MDPI
St. Alban-Anlage 66
4052 Basel, Switzerland

This is a reprint of articles from the Special Issue published online in the open access journal *Diagnostics* (ISSN 2075-4418) (available at: www.mdpi.com/journal/diagnostics/special_issues/ Endometriosis_Diagnosis).

For citation purposes, cite each article independently as indicated on the article page online and as indicated below:

LastName, A.A.; LastName, B.B.; LastName, C.C. Article Title. *Journal Name* **Year**, *Volume Number*, Page Range.

ISBN 978-3-0365-2801-4 (Hbk)
ISBN 978-3-0365-2800-7 (PDF)

© 2022 by the authors. Articles in this book are Open Access and distributed under the Creative Commons Attribution (CC BY) license, which allows users to download, copy and build upon published articles, as long as the author and publisher are properly credited, which ensures maximum dissemination and a wider impact of our publications.

The book as a whole is distributed by MDPI under the terms and conditions of the Creative Commons license CC BY-NC-ND.

Contents

About the Editor vii

Marco Scioscia, Bruna A. Virgilio, Antonio Simone Laganà, Tommaso Bernardini, Nicola Fattizzi, Manuela Neri and Stefano Guerriero
Differential Diagnosis of Endometriosis by Ultrasound: A Rising Challenge
Reprinted from: *Diagnostics* 2020, 10, 848, doi:10.3390/diagnostics10100848 1

Gábor Szabó, István Madár, Attila Bokor and János Rigó
Transvaginal Strain Elastosonography May Help in the Differential Diagnosis of Endometriosis?
Reprinted from: *Diagnostics* 2021, 11, 100, doi:10.3390/diagnostics11010100 17

Marco Scioscia, Antonio Simone Laganà, Giuseppe Caringella and Stefano Guerriero
Transvaginal Strain Elastosonography in the Differential Diagnosis of Rectal Endometriosis: Some Potentials and Limits
Reprinted from: *Diagnostics* 2021, 11, 99, doi:10.3390/diagnostics11010099 21

Fabio Barra, Ennio Biscaldi, Carolina Scala, Antonio Simone Laganà, Valerio Gaetano Vellone, Cesare Stabilini, Fabio Ghezzi and Simone Ferrero
A Prospective Study Comparing Three-Dimensional Rectal Water Contrast Transvaginal Ultrasonography and Computed Tomographic Colonography in the Diagnosis of Rectosigmoid Endometriosis
Reprinted from: *Diagnostics* 2020, 10, 252, doi:10.3390/diagnostics10040252 25

Jessica Ottolina, Ludovica Bartiromo, Carolina Dolci, Noemi Salmeri, Matteo Schimberni, Roberta Villanacci, Paola Viganò and Massimo Candiani
Assessment of Coagulation Parameters in Women Affected by Endometriosis: Validation Study and Systematic Review of the Literature
Reprinted from: *Diagnostics* 2020, 10, 567, doi:10.3390/diagnostics10080567 41

Carolina Filipchiuk, Antonio Simone Laganà, Rubia Beteli, Tatiana Guida Ponce, Denise Maria Christofolini, Camila Martins Trevisan, Fernando Luiz Affonso Fonseca, Caio Parente Barbosa and Bianca Bianco
BIRC5/Survivin Expression as a Non-Invasive Biomarker of Endometriosis
Reprinted from: *Diagnostics* 2020, 10, 533, doi:10.3390/diagnostics10080533 59

Zeenat Mirza and Umama A. Abdel-dayem
Uncovering Potential Roles of Differentially Expressed Genes, Upstream Regulators, and Canonical Pathways in Endometriosis Using an In Silico Genomics Approach
Reprinted from: *Diagnostics* 2020, 10, 416, doi:10.3390/diagnostics10060416 69

Camila Hernandes, Paola Silveira, Aline Fernanda Rodrigues Sereia, Ana Paula Christoff, Helen Mendes, Luiz Felipe Valter de Oliveira and Sergio Podgaec
Microbiome Profile of Deep Endometriosis Patients: Comparison of Vaginal Fluid, Endometrium and Lesion
Reprinted from: *Diagnostics* 2020, 10, 163, doi:10.3390/diagnostics10030163 85

Cristina Secosan, Ligia Balulescu, Simona Brasoveanu, Oana Balint, Paul Pirtea, Grigoraș Dorin and Laurentiu Pirtea
Endometriosis in Menopause—Renewed Attention on a Controversial Disease
Reprinted from: *Diagnostics* 2020, 10, 134, doi:10.3390/diagnostics10030134 97

Ana M. Sanchez, Luca Pagliardini, Greta C. Cermisoni, Laura Privitera, Sofia Makieva, Alessandra Alteri, Laura Corti, Elisa Rabellotti, Massimo Candiani and Paola Viganò
Does Endometriosis Influence the Embryo Quality and/or Development? Insights from a Large Retrospective Matched Cohort Study
Reprinted from: *Diagnostics* **2020**, *10*, 83, doi:10.3390/diagnostics10020083 . . . . **109**

About the Editor

Antonio Simone Laganà

Medical Doctor at the Department of Obstetrics and Gynecology, "Filippo Del Ponte" Hospital, University of Insubria, Varese, Italy.

Antonio Simone Laganà was born in Reggio Calabria (Italy) on 8th May 1986. He is Deputy of the Special Interest Group for Endometriosis & Endometrial Disorders (SIGEED) of the European Society of Human Reproduction and Embryology (ESHRE) and Ambassador of the World Endometriosis Society (WES).

His research interests include endometriosis, reproductive immunology, infertility, gynaecological endocrinology, laparoscopy, and hysteroscopy. He is the author of more than 300 papers published in PubMed-indexed international peer-reviewed journals, and his presence is often requested as an invited speaker at international congresses. He is currently an editor of high-impact journals, including Scientific Reports, PLOS One, Journal of Minimally Invasive Gynecology, Journal of Ovarian Research, Gynecologic and Obstetric Investigation, and many others. He is habilitated as Associate Professor in Italy for Gynecology and Obstetrics.

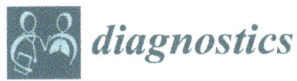

Review

Differential Diagnosis of Endometriosis by Ultrasound: A Rising Challenge

Marco Scioscia [1], Bruna A. Virgilio [1], Antonio Simone Laganà [2,*], Tommaso Bernardini [1], Nicola Fattizzi [1], Manuela Neri [3,4] and Stefano Guerriero [3,4]

1. Department of Obstetrics and Gynecology, Policlinico Hospital, 35031 Abano Terme, PD, Italy; marcoscioscia@gmail.com (M.S.); bruna81@tiscali.it (B.A.V.); tbernardini@casacura.it (T.B.); nfattizzi@casacura.it (N.F.)
2. Department of Obstetrics and Gynecology, "Filippo Del Ponte" Hospital, University of Insubria, 21100 Varese, VA, Italy
3. Obstetrics and Gynecology, University of Cagliari, 09124 Cagliari, CA, Italy; manu.neri11@hotmail.it (M.N.); gineca.sguerriero@tiscali.it (S.G.)
4. Department of Obstetrics and Gynecology, Azienda Ospedaliero Universitaria, Policlinico Universitario Duilio Casula, 09045 Monserrato, CA, Italy
* Correspondence: antoniosimone.lagana@uninsubria.it

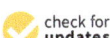

Received: 6 October 2020; Accepted: 15 October 2020; Published: 20 October 2020

Abstract: Ultrasound is an effective tool to detect and characterize endometriosis lesions. Variances in endometriosis lesions' appearance and distorted anatomy secondary to adhesions and fibrosis present as major difficulties during the complete sonographic evaluation of pelvic endometriosis. Currently, differential diagnosis of endometriosis to distinguish it from other diseases represents the hardest challenge and affects subsequent treatment. Several gynecological and non-gynecological conditions can mimic deep-infiltrating endometriosis. For example, abdominopelvic endometriosis may present as atypical lesions by ultrasound. Here, we present an overview of benign and malignant diseases that may resemble endometriosis of the internal genitalia, bowels, bladder, ureter, peritoneum, retroperitoneum, as well as less common locations. An accurate diagnosis of endometriosis has significant clinical impact and is important for appropriate treatment.

Keywords: endometriosis; adenomyosis; bowel; rectum; ovary; bladder; ureter; abdominal wall; vagina

1. Introduction

Endometriosis is a common, chronic, and debilitating gynecological condition that affects between 5–15% of women within their reproductive ages [1,2]. It is characterized by the growth of tissue that mimics endometrial tissue and exhibits the same responses to hormonal changes [1]. However, this abnormal tissue growth occurs outside the uterus, usually on other organs inside the pelvis and abdominal cavity, thus creating endometriosis implants. These endometriosis implants lead to local inflammatory reactions that promote fibrosis and adhesion formation, which create resistance between organs and may result in an altered pelvic anatomy [3]. This cascade of events often causes menstrual and/or chronic pelvic pain, infertility, or malfunction of the affected abdominopelvic organs [1].

In the past decades, ultrasound has become a valuable tool to accompany pelvic bimanual examinations. Currently, both methods are used for the first-line examination and diagnosis of endometriosis [4]. When a patient presents with persistent symptoms of suspected endometriosis, a comprehensive and detailed evaluation of the pelvis by ultrasound is usually prescribed. However, the accuracy of the ultrasound in detecting deep-infiltrating endometriosis depends on the experience of the sonographer. Variances in endometriosis lesion appearance and distorted anatomy secondary to adhesions and fibrosis present as major difficulties during the complete sonographic evaluation of pelvic endometriosis [5].

Therefore, a trained ultrasound operator is needed to detect most of the endometriosis lesions, and is required to make sound judgments and to plan the appropriate treatment [5,6]. It is also important for expert evaluations to include a differential diagnosis (DD) of endometriosis to exclude all other abdominopelvic diseases. Although misdiagnoses represent a small number of cases with unknown prevalence (Figure 1), the clinical impact of a DD is great because the appropriate treatment largely varies based on the diagnosis.

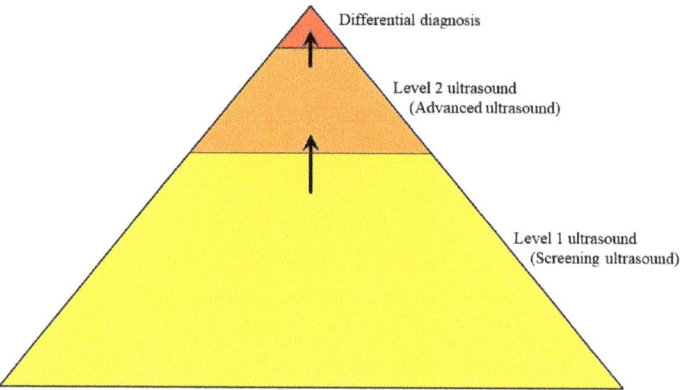

Figure 1. A pyramid chart that represents the distribution of ultrasound scans for endometriosis according to complexity. Although differential diagnosis must be considered in each exam, the number of cases where it makes a difference is relatively small, although it is fundamental.

2. What a Comprehensive Ultrasound for Endometriosis Should Investigate

Traditionally, a routine pelvic ultrasound only evaluates uterine and ovarian lesions, which leads to the detection of elementary lesions, such as endometriomas [7]. However, the evaluation should include the anterior and posterior pelvic compartments to assess the mobility of pelvic organs [7–10] and to improve the assessment of endometriosis, as suggested by the International Deep Endometriosis Analysis (IDEA) consensus [11]. The use of a systematic ultrasound approach can enhance the detection of different endometriosis locations within the pelvis [12–14], with a detection rate that is similar to that of magnetic resonance [15,16].

Endometriosis can extend to organs other than internal genitalia, such as the bowels, bladder [1,16], and retroperitoneal structures (e.g., ureters, parametria, nerves) [17], which significantly complicates the ultrasound evaluation [18]. Although all these locations appear similar on an ultrasound (nodular, sometimes flat, hypoechoic lesions with the absence of colored Doppler spots), and they present specific features according to the organ or tissue involved. In fact, deep-infiltrating endometriosis (DIE) of hollow organs induces a retraction of margins with a subsequent irregular profile of both external and internal surfaces (i.e., bladder, bowels, and vagina), whereas DIE of dense organs (i.e., peritoneal and retroperitoneal organs) maintains a nodular hypoechoic structure [11]. Less frequently, some lesions may display vascularity with small cysts (i.e., bladder; Figure 2). Cystic endometriosis of retroperitoneal organs is a rare event that mainly occurs in patients with a history of pelvic surgery (Figure 3).

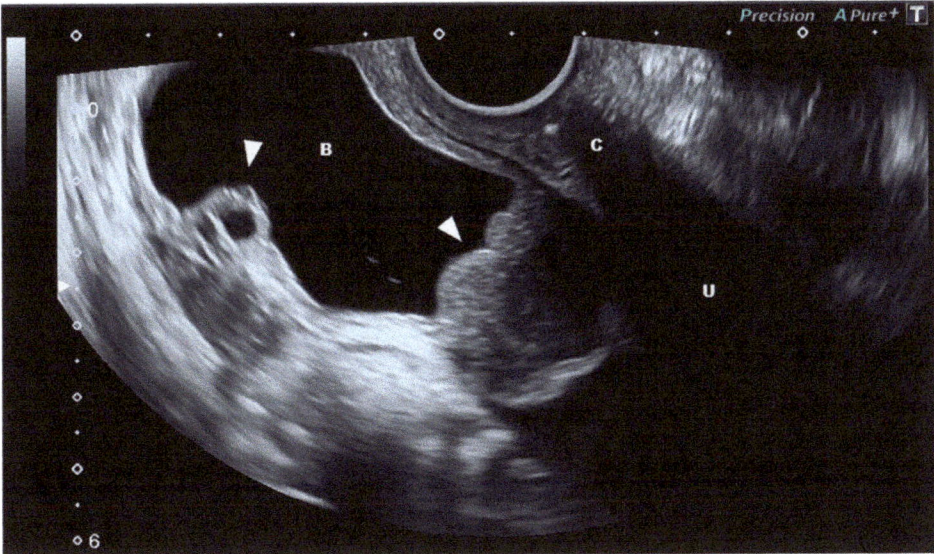

Figure 2. Bifocal endometriosis of the bladder (arrow). The two lesions present different characteristics as the one on the right-hand side presents a typical solid aspect while the left one is a cystic endometriosis location. Abbreviations: B, bladder; C, cervix; U, uterus.

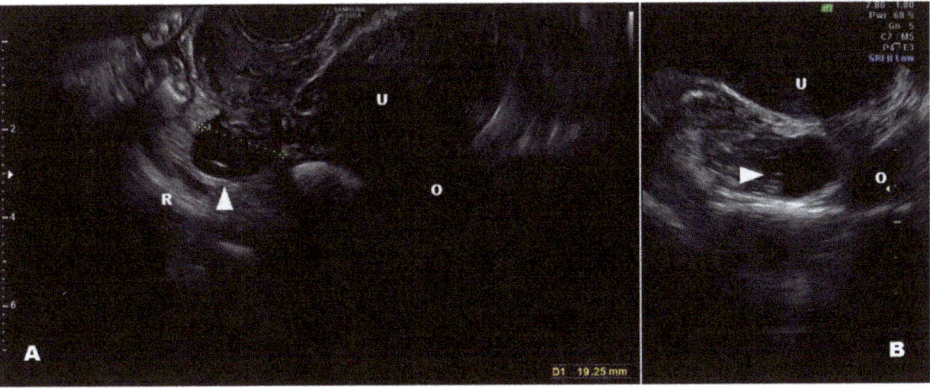

Figure 3. Cystic endometriosis (arrow) of the retroperitoneum in two patients on medical therapy with previous pelvic surgery for endometriosis. (**A**) shows an endometriosis cyst of the rectovaginal septum and (**B**) shows a cyst of the mesometrium. Abbreviations: U, uterus; R, rectum; O, Ovary.

3. Sonographic Differential Diagnosis

During a comprehensive evaluation, the sonographer should be able to correctly identify all significant endometriosis lesions, the presence of other benign diseases (i.e., fibroids, uterine malformations, etc.), and any suspected malignancies. It is also important that the DD includes examination for adenomyosis [12,19–21] and endometrioma [22,23]. It is far more difficult for gynecologists to identify and characterize diseases of organs other than the internal genitalia. However, the ultrasound operator must be competent in identifying not only normal and altered pelvic anatomy due to endometriosis and other gynecological diseases, but also other diseases that are typically identified by other specialists (e.g., radiologist, gastroenterologist, urologist). Furthermore, gynecologists also have to consider that the presence of endometriosis does not exclude other clinical conditions that may require further evaluation by another specialist.

Several gynecological and non-gynecological conditions can mimic DIE, which are summarized in Table 1. In some cases, clinical signs can help differentiate diseases even when a pelvic bimanual examination is suggestive of endometriosis. Several studies have demonstrated the possibility of a DD of endometriosis lesions with benign (e.g., adenomyoma vs. myoma or endometrioma vs. other cysts) [19,22,24–26] and malignant genital diseases (e.g., ovarian cancer) [26,27].

Table 1. Endometriosis possible anatomic locations, anatomical features, and differential diagnosis.

Anatomic Locations	Anatomical Aspect	Possible Differential Diagnosis
Internal genitalia		
Ovary	Cystic	Hemorrhagic corpus luteus Hemorrhagic cyst Dermoid cyst Tubovarian abscess Mucinous cystoadenoma Ovarian cystic adenomyoma Malignancy
Tube	Cystic	Tubovarian abscess
Uterus (adenomyosis)	Focal, solid (buds)	Endometrial malignancy
	Solid adenomyoma	Non-encapsulated myomas
	Cystic adenomyoma	Myomas with cystic degeneration/necrosis Suspected sarcoma/STUMP
Vagina	Solid nodulus	Cervical malignancy Vaginal malignancy
	Cystic	Benign vaginal cyst
Peritoneum		
Broad anterior/posterior ligament	Solid	Peritoneal carcinomatosis
Douglas pouch	Solid	Peritoneal carcinomatosis Advanced cervical malignancy
Prevesical peritoneum	Solid	Post-cesarean adhesions Peritoneal carcinomatosis Advanced cervical malignancy
Uterosacral ligaments	Solid	Peritoneal carcinomatosis Advanced cervical malignancy
Round ligaments	Solid	Peritoneal carcinomatosis Advanced endometrial malignancy
Retroperitoneal tissues		
Paracervix/parametrium	Solid	Advanced cervical malignancy
Mesometrium	Solid	Pedunculated infraligamentary fibroid Ovarian malignancy
	Cystic	Varicocele

Table 1. Cont.

Anatomic Locations	Anatomical Aspect	Possible Differential Diagnosis
Mesorectum	Solid	Colonic malignancy Downward dislocated appendix
	Cystic	Retrorectal dermoid cyst
Presacral space	Cystic	Tarlov cyst Ganglioneuroma
Vesicovaginal septum	Solid	Bladder malignancy
Bowel		
Rectosigmoid	Solid	Colonic polyp Diverticulosis Colonic malignancy
Caecum and appendix	Solid	Appendicitis Appendiceal tumors
Ileum	Solid	Malignancy
Urinary tract		
Bladder	Solid	Bladder malignancy Cervical malignancy Uterine leiomyomas/adenomyomas Hypertrophic traumatic bladder
	Cystic	Bladder malignancy Intravesical ureterocele Small bowel attached to the prevesical peritoneum
Ureter	Solid	Ureteric stone
External genitalia		
Perineum	Solid	Postpatum scar Chron disease
Mons pubis	Solid	Abscess Hematoma Muscular strain
Abdominal wall		
Umbilicus	Solid	Omphalitis Umbilical granuloma
Abdominal muscle	Solid	Strain Benign tumor (desmoid)
	Cystic	Hematoma
Inguinal canal	Solid	Complete small hernia

3.1. Internal Genitalia

The ovary is the most common site of endometriosis (Table 1). Additionally, the "typical" endometrioma in premenopausal women is the easiest to identify by ultrasound due to its specific characteristics (e.g., unilocular cysts with ground-glass echogenicity of the fluid content, polar clot/debris, and poor vascularization on color Doppler evaluation) [28,29]. This should be differentiated by hemorrhagic corpora lutea especially when fine strands of fibrin are seen in the fluid content of the cyst, through the evidence of rich peripheral vascularization and its transient nature. Sometimes a correct diagnosis is not easy, especially in the presence of multiple cysts, because it can be very difficult to distinguish an endometrioma from other adnexal masses, such as some dermoid cysts, hemorrhagic cysts, tubovarian abscesses, mucinous cystadenomas, or ovarian cystic adenomyomas [24–26]. The presence of intracystic vascularization certainly poses doubts about malignancy (e.g., borderline tumor, endometrioid cancer) [23] also because 1% of the masses presumed to be endometriomas are malignant [30]. Furthermore, the ultrasound characteristics of pre- and postmenopausal endometriomas differ. Postmenopausal endometriomas are less frequently unilocular and are less likely to have ground-glass content; however, those with typical ground-glass content have a high risk of malignancy [28].

Superficial endometriosis of the fallopian tubes is undetectable, but it can be suspected by the presence of a tubovarian complex with tube dilatation at the location of the endometriomas. Sonographic diagnosis of tubovarian abscesses is not easy in such cases, but the clinical presentations of tube wall edema and positive color/power Doppler intensities are suggestive [31], regardless of the presence of an endometrioma (abscess superimposed to the endometriosis tubovarian complex). Solid localizations of the fallopian tubes are certainly difficult to detect but they do not require a DD in the presence of other pelvic endometriosis lesions.

Adenomyosis is characterized by an altered junctional zone with an area that is isoechoic to the endometrial tissue (for the deepening of ectopic endometrial glands and stroma), and its ultrasound classification has been well described [19,32]. It can often present as an irregularity of the junctional zone (e.g., echogenic subendometrial lines and buds, an interrupted junctional zone) with or without myometrial cystic lesions, which appear either as focal or diffuse lesions or as adenomyomas. Solid lesions, which are referred to as buds, that originate from the endometrium must be differentiated from non-endophytic endometrial cancers, such as uterine clear-cell carcinoma and uterine papillary serous carcinoma. Buds do not develop from endometrial hyperplasia, but instead they arise from an atrophic endometrium [33]. The age of onset, which largely overlaps [34], clinical presentation [35], and endometrial thickness (women with symptomatic adenomyosis or perimenopausal menstrual alterations are often on hormonal therapy) may not help in the DD; however, the myometrial vascularization may provide some clues. In adenomyosis cases, the vessel distribution (i.e., arcuate, radial, and basal arteries) within the myometrium and the lesion is not altered [19,32], whereas the neoangiogenesis that occurs in tumoral lesions is detected by color/power Doppler and the identification of aberrant vessels, even in cases of endometrial cancer in which the endometrium does not appear particularly irregular [36].

Adenomyomas are defined as benign tumors that include components derived from endometrial glands, stroma, muscular cells, and fibrosis [20]. These lesions are mostly found within the myometrium, and their sonographic characteristics resemble those of myomas. Nevertheless, in some cases they can be differentiated from myomas [21]. The correct preoperative diagnosis between myomas and adenomyomas is of key importance for surgeons because the surgical removal of adenomyomas is very difficult, if not impossible. The ultrasound characteristics of adenomyomas have been reported [12,19], and their DD mainly consists of the absence of both the pseudocapsule and vascularization compared with that of myomas. In fact, non-encapsulated myomas that lack the typical refraction at the mass border maintain the typical circumferential vascularization of fibroids, whereas adenomyomas exhibit an anatomical myometrial pattern of vessels (i.e., arcuate, radial, and basal arteries). Lacunas are not necessarily a sign of adenomyomas because uterine fibroids may exhibit cystic degeneration secondary to a limited blood supply. In fact, the thick hyperechoic wall of the cystic glands of adenomyomas is poorly represented during hormonal therapy, thus a clear DD may not be possible. Clinical symptoms may support the findings of the sonographic examination because uterine myomas with cystic degeneration are poorly symptomatic, unless they are submucosal. However, adenomyomas may present with abnormal uterine bleeding and periodic pain during ovulation and menstruations. In cases of uterine masses with strong vascularity, usually hypervascular myomas, a DD that includes adenomyosis, occult degeneration (leiomyosarcoma or smooth uterine muscle of uncertain malignant potential [STUMP]), or a benign fibroid is not possible [21].

Endometriosis of the vagina occurs in approximately 12% of women with revised American Society for Reproductive Medicine (rASRM) stage IV endometriosis [17]. It presents as a nodular thickening of the vaginal wall that causes pain under a gentle pressure with the probe [37] and that does not modify with probe compression [22]. It infiltrates the recto-vaginal septum, usually in the posterior or lateral-posterior upper third of the vagina, and it presents as a hypoechoic lesion with a negative/minimal color Doppler signaling. Its DD must include advanced cervical cancer with vaginal infiltration. The normal appearance of the uterine cervix with different vascularization as well as symptoms after intercourse (endometriosis is associated to dyspareunia, whereas cervical cancer is associated with postcoital bleeding) can lead to a correct diagnosis. A DD that includes rare tumors, such as those of primary vaginal cancer, is mainly clinical because of its clinical appearance and the age of diagnosis (more frequent in postmenopausal women).

Endometriosis of the vagina rarely presents as cystic and is usually a part of a larger solid nodule. Vaginal cysts have been reported to occur in approximately 1% of all women, and they are located in the anterolateral vaginal wall [38]. These cysts are asymptomatic remnants of the Wolffian duct and present as regular hypo- or anechoic cysts. Less frequently, they can be located on the posterolateral vaginal wall within vaginal scars (i.e., episiotomy and birth lacerations). The key aspects for a DD are the location (endometriosis is always on the posterior vaginal wall) and the absence of tenderness.

3.2. Peritoneal and Retroperitoneal Endometriosis Lesions

The pelvic peritoneum is almost always involved in advanced-stage endometriosis [3,17]. The typical appearance is a nodular thickening of the peritoneum, which is sometimes nodular or flat, like a plaque (this is very often found beneath the ovary on the ovarian fossa), and hypoechoic with negative color Doppler signaling. These lesions may grow inward into tissues from a superficial site of origin, deepening further into the mesometrium (endophytic growth) and reaching subperitoneal structures, such as ligaments (e.g., uterosacral and round), ureters, and superficial nerves (e.g., hypogastric nerve). The DD includes peritoneal carcinomatosis that presents as nodular or sheet-like, exophytic, hypoechoic, vascularized structures and is almost always associated with ascites [39].

The peritoneum over the uterus and bladder can be clearly evaluated by a transvaginal scan with an unemptied bladder, and any lesions with enough thickness (nodule) can be identified [40]. Although superficial, plain lesions cannot be detected, alterations in the peritoneal profile due to retractive fibrosis and adhesions have sometimes been reported [22]. The presence of adhesions in prevesical peritoneum due to a cesarean section with the absence of the uterine sliding sign are often misleading and impossible to differentiate from endometriosis. The two clinical conditions (adhesions and endometriosis) can coexist, and it is important to evaluate if a peritoneal lesion of endometriosis deepens into the vesicovaginal septum to the bladder.

Retroperitoneal endometriosis near the uterus (i.e., paracervical and parametrial) is common [17,41], and ultrasound is a valid tool to identify these lesions [11,42–45]. A DD that includes the spread of cervical cancer warrants attention [46]. Endometriosis of the broad posterior ligaments may infiltrate deeply into the mesometrium and paracervical tissues, reaching organs, such as the ureter [47], and appearing as a solid nodule in most cases. Retroperitoneal cystic endometriosis is not very common (Figure 3B), and it typically occurs in women who previously had pelvic surgery for endometriosis. However, it should be differentiated from a pelvic varicocele. A misplaced appendix may be easily confused with endometriosis of the mesorectum, which is usually superficial and presents as a peritoneal implant of endometriosis (Figure 4) [48]. Cystic endometriosis beneath the rectum is very rare [49] compared with benign cysts of sacral nerve roots.

3.3. The Bowels

Colonic endometriosis is not a rare condition. It affects 37% of women with severe endometriosis [13], and its correct diagnosis is essential for the proper planning of treatment [15,48,50,51]. Recently, the ultrasound detection rate of endometriosis foci of the bowels has increased, exhibiting both high sensitivity and specificity [46,52]. Additionally, its accuracy is as high as other imaging techniques, such as magnetic resonance, rectal endoscopy sonography, and double contrast barium enema [11,12,15,53]. Bowel lesions can present as different shapes; however, they exhibit an anechoic appearance without posterior enhancement, they can invade the bowel lumen, and they can have digitiform, irregular, or smooth limits. The sliding sign with the uterus and near organs is often negative because the nodule may involve the Douglas pouch or the uterosacral ligaments, or it can be attached to the posterior wall of the uterus.

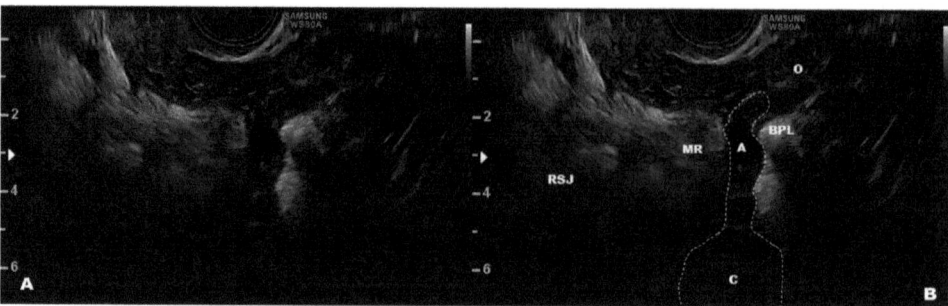

Figure 4. Appendix dislocated downward and attached to the ovary that may mimic mesorectal endometriosis. (**A**,**B**) show the clean and the labelled image. Abbreviations: A, appendix; O, Ovary; BPL, broad posterior ligament; C, caecum; MR, mesorectum; RSJ, rectosigmoid junction.

The DD of bowel endometriosis using ultrasound is particularly challenging for gynecologists who are not used to examining lesions other than those of endometriosis. In some cases, bowel disease may resemble endometriosis, and the DD is more difficult [54]. It is important to note that rectosigmoid endometriosis always involves the anterior or the lateral rectosigmoid wall and never the posterior wall that is directed toward the mesorectum/mesosigmoid [54]. The most common bowel diseases that can be mistaken for endometriosis include appendicitis, appendiceal tumors [48], colonic polyps, diverticulosis, and colonic malignancy [54]. Specific factors of the internal surface of the gut should be considered during a DD, such as colonic polyps and malignancies. As we reported in a previous article [54], colon cancer growths typically extend outward and reach the serosa, whereas endometriosis lesions grow inward. A transrectal ultrasound with a radial probe that scans the entire 360 degrees of the rectal lumen is a useful tool to detect and confirm the presence of polyps or malignancies; however, a colonoscopy remains the gold standard for diagnosis. In advanced-stage rectal cancer, there may be infiltration of the entire bowel wall, but the presence of specific symptoms (e.g., rectal bleeding, unexplained weight loss, gas pains or cramps) may help with the correct diagnosis.

It may also be difficult to distinguish bowel endometriosis from colonic diverticula [54]. Diverticula are mainly characterized as outward growths on a thick bowel wall with hyperechoic content, whereas endometriosis is endophytic and hypoechoic. The imaging may even be more complex if inflammation occurs within a closed diverticular abscess. In this case, an undefined oval mass that is growing outward beyond the bowel surface may be identified. Additionally, a transverse section may exhibit intense Doppler positivity in acute diverticulitis. Clinical symptoms (e.g., constant abdominal tenderness, nausea and vomiting, and pyrexia) and inflammatory blood tests may support the sonographic findings and lead to the correct diagnosis and treatment.

3.4. The Bladder and Ureter

Urinary tract endometriosis occurs in 0.3–12% of women with endometriosis [55,56], with an incidence of 43% in women with stage IV endometriosis [17]. Endometriosis of the muscularis propria of the bladder and the ureters are the rarest conditions, with incidences of 4.3% and 9.5%, respectively [17]. The bladder wall can be examined by ultrasound because it is surrounded by a low-echogenic tissue (i.e., perivesical loose connective tissue) and the peritoneum, which appears as a hyperechoic line. In most cases, a hypoechoic lesion that alters the profile of the peritoneum of the bladder and infiltrates into the detrusor muscle indicates bladder endometriosis and originates from uterine adenomyosis [50]. Endometriosis of the bladder is often symptomatic (e.g., urgency, frequency, and pain on passing urine, which worsen days before and during menstruation, and recurrent urinary tract infections) and appears as a consistently solid mass that involves the prevesical space, the serosa (adventitia), and the detrusor muscle, sometimes up to the urothelium [22,42,57]. These lesions always involve the bladder dome on the sagittal plane, and sometimes the nodule may also extend laterally. Additionally, they exhibit color Doppler positivity. The vascularity of these lesions may suggest a malignant origin of the nodule; however, only advanced-stage cancer (either a bladder or cervical carcinoma) invades the prevesical peritoneum. Furthermore, bladder cancer is typically found in postmenopausal women and originates from the internal surface (urothelium) of the lateral wall of the bladder. In cases of advanced-stage cervical cancer, the lesion clearly involves the cervix and quite often the lateral parametrial and paracervical tissues [50,58]. Endometriosis of the bladder may present some uncommon features, such as cystic lesions and multifocal endometriosis. In such cases, it is very difficult to differentiate from bladder cancer that may be both cystic and multifocal [59,60]. Vesical cancer usually presents as a solid papillary mass that projects into the bladder, with a normal thickness of the bladder wall at the site of the lesion [60]. Nevertheless, large carcinomas may exhibit anechoic cystic degeneration within the mass and infiltration of the detrusor muscle [60]. Color Doppler imaging is not useful for this condition because cystic endometriosis of the bladder usually shows no vascularization. When making the DD, the facts that bladder carcinomas typically occur in elderly women and that urinary cytology is the simplest, less-invasive, and least expensive method to obtain a correct diagnosis warrants consideration [50].

We recently reviewed the DD of urinary tract endometriosis [50]. The DD may sometimes be difficult due to the presence of external masses that encroach the bladder dome (i.e., uterine fibroids or an attached small bowel from a previous surgery, such as a cesarean section), an intravesical ureterocele that may resemble deep lesions of endometriosis, or hypertrophic areas of the bladder wall due to a chronic, complete cystocele and recurrent cystitis [50]. In such cases, although bladder endometriosis very often appears as an endophytic lesion, it may sometimes appear flat and may be confused with hypertrophic areas due to chronic mechanical trauma (cystocele) or recurrent cystitis (Figure 5).

Endometriosis of the ureter affects the pelvic segment of the organ as a deepening of foci of the posterior broad ligament. Endometrial tissue may only invade the outer adventitia (extrinsic type) or the mucosal and/or muscular layers of the ureter (intrinsic type) [22,61]. It presents as a nodule along the course of the ureter that causes a dilatation of the ureteral tract proximal to the stenosis. The dilated ureter appears as a blood vessel in the parametrial tissue with negative color Doppler signaling and evidence of peristalsis [47], which is also often associated with hydronephrosis. The presence of ureteric calculi, which cause intense symptoms and appear as solid echogenic masses often with dilatation of the proximal part of the ureter, must be excluded [50].

3.5. Uncommon Endometriosis Locations

Uncommon locations of endometriosis are difficult to detect, and the accuracy of the ultrasound may be significantly reduced due to an inexperienced operator [62]. Endometriosis of the external genitalia (e.g., the perineum and mons pubis) may be easily confused with other conditions (i.e., abscesses, genital Crohn's disease, skin trauma/swollen lesions, and hematomas) [63,64] because it may originate from abdominal wall lesions (i.e., muscular strains, heparin hematomas, muscular tumors, and hernias). In such cases, patient history in addition to the ultrasound findings is useful for identification of any conditions that resemble endometriosis [65–67]. The rarest sites of endometriosis include lesions of the liver, pancreas, kidney, and gallbladder. Hepatic endometriosis appears as superficial hypoechoic lesions and may mimic an abscess, a hematoma, an angioma, or malignancy [62].

Endometriosis of pancreas, kidney, and gallbladder show hypoechoic lesions that can be seen by ultrasound and they require a second evaluation by computerized tomography or magnetic resonance imaging [62]. These lesions do not present pathognomonic features that may differentiate endometriosis from malignancy or adenomas, so the definitive diagnosis relies on histology only [62].

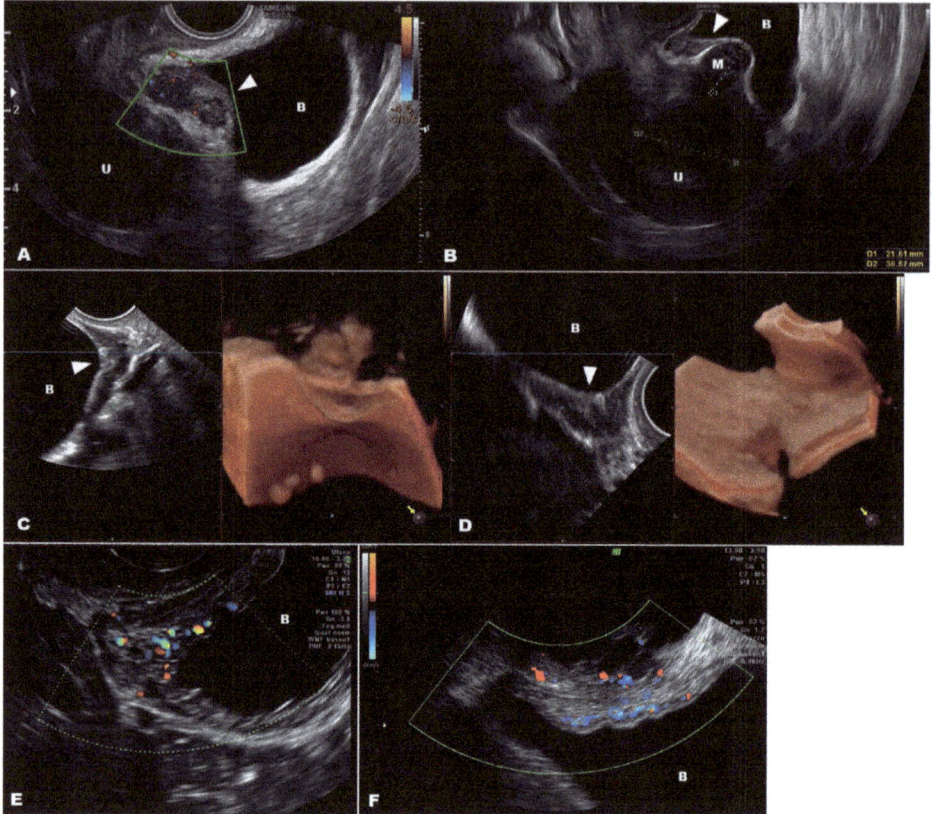

Figure 5. A typical endometriosis nodule (arrow) of the bladder (**A**); figure (**B**) shows a flat nodule of endometriosis (arrow) with a subserosal myoma that distorts the bladder dome; a flat endometriosis nodule (arrow) of the bladder that can be seen at 3D ultrasound only when cut (**C**) while the internal surface of the bladder appears regular (**D**); figure (**E**) shows a thick bladder wall due to cystocele and figure (**F**) in case of recurrent cystitis. Abbreviations: U, uterus; B, bladder; M, myoma.

4. Conclusions

The accuracy of ultrasound for the diagnosis of pelvic endometriosis has greatly improved over recent years, and it is widely regarded as the first-line diagnostic tool, despite a significant interobserver variability has been reported [68]. Certainly, the identification of extra-genitalia lesions requires a specific training [69]; however, ongoing practice is necessary to acquire and maintain competence [70].

DD by ultrasound for patients who have been referred for endometriosis may result in the detection of other gynecological diseases; therefore, it is important to consider other conditions when unusual lesions are detected. A skilled operator is key because his mental reconstruction of the distorted anatomy is necessary to correctly localize and evaluate the lesion of interest. Additional knowledge of the ultrasound appearances of lesions that do not occur within the reproductive system is needed to make a correct diagnosis. however, in such cases, further examinations should be required, or patients should be referred to other experts/specialists. A specific hands-on training for making DDs is not possible, but theoretical courses and off-line scanning sessions for sonographers with experience in gynecological and endometriosis ultrasound help to improve their background and may result in more accurate diagnoses.

Author Contributions: Conceptualization, M.S. and B.A.V.; methodology, S.G.; data curation, M.S., B.A.V., and T.B.; writing—original draft preparation, M.S.; writing—review and editing, A.S.L., N.F., and M.N.; visualization, M.S.; supervision, S.G. All authors have read and agreed to the published version of the manuscript.

Funding: This research received no external funding.

Conflicts of Interest: The authors declare no conflict of interest.

References

1. Zondervan, K.T.; Becker, C.M.; Missmer, S.A. Endometriosis. *N. Engl. J. Med.* **2020**, *382*, 1244–1256. [CrossRef] [PubMed]
2. Nnoaham, K.E.; Hummelshoj, L.; Webster, P.; d'Hooghe, T.; de Cicco Nardone, F.; de Cicco Nardone, C.; Jenkinson, C.; Kennedy, S.H.; Zondervan, K.T. World Endometriosis Research Foundation Global Study of Women's Health consortium Impact of endometriosis on quality of life and work productivity: A multicenter study across ten countries. *Fertil. Steril.* **2011**, *96*, 366373.e8. [CrossRef]
3. Burney, R.O.; Giudice, L.C. Pathogenesis and pathophysiology of endometriosis. *Fertil. Steril.* **2012**, *98*, 511–519. [CrossRef] [PubMed]
4. Dunselman, G.A.J.; Vermeulen, N.; Becker, C.; Calhaz-Jorge, C.; D'Hooghe, T.; De Bie, B.; Heikinheimo, O.; Horne, A.W.; Kiesel, L.; Nap, A.; et al. ESHRE guideline: Management of women with endometriosis. *Hum. Reprod.* **2014**, *29*, 400–412. [CrossRef] [PubMed]
5. Schliep, K.; Chen, Z.; Stanford, J.; Xie, Y.; Mumford, S.; Hammoud, A.; Boiman Johnstone, E.; Dorais, J.; Varner, M.; Buck Louis, G.; et al. Endometriosis diagnosis and staging by operating surgeon and expert review using multiple diagnostic tools: An inter-rater agreement study. *BJOG Int. J. Obstet. Gynecol.* **2017**, *124*, 220–229. [CrossRef] [PubMed]
6. Chapron, C.; Marcellin, L.; Borghese, B.; Santulli, P. Rethinking mechanisms, diagnosis and management of endometriosis. *Nat. Rev. Endocrinol.* **2019**, *15*, 666–682. [CrossRef] [PubMed]
7. Collins, B.G.; Ankola, A.; Gola, S.; McGillen, K.L. Transvaginal US of Endometriosis: Looking Beyond the Endometrioma with a Dedicated Protocol. *Radiographics* **2019**, *39*, 1549–1568. [CrossRef]
8. Piessens, S.; Edwards, A. Sonographic Evaluation for Endometriosis in Routine Pelvic Ultrasound. *J. Minim. Invasive Gynecol.* **2020**, *27*, 265–266. [CrossRef] [PubMed]
9. Fraser, M.A.; Agarwal, S.; Chen, I.; Singh, S.S. Routine vs. expert-guided transvaginal ultrasound in the diagnosis of endometriosis: A retrospective review. *Abdom. Imaging* **2015**, *40*, 587–594. [CrossRef]
10. Fratelli, N.; Scioscia, M.; Bassi, E.; Musola, M.; Minelli, L.; Trivella, G. Transvaginal sonography for preoperative assessment of deep endometriosis. *J. Clin. Ultrasound* **2013**, *41*, 69–75. [CrossRef]
11. Guerriero, S.; Condous, G.; van den Bosch, T.; Valentin, L.; Leone, F.P.G.; Van Schoubroeck, D.; Exacoustos, C.; Installé, A.J.F.; Martins, W.P.; Abrao, M.S.; et al. Systematic approach to sonographic evaluation of the pelvis in women with suspected endometriosis, including terms, definitions and measurements: A consensus opinion from the International Deep Endometriosis Analysis (IDEA) group. *Ultrasound Obstet. Gynecol.* **2016**, *48*, 318–332. [CrossRef] [PubMed]
12. Van den Bosch, T.; Van Schoubroeck, D. Ultrasound diagnosis of endometriosis and adenomyosis: State of the art. *Best Pract. Res. Clin. Obstet. Gynaecol.* **2018**, *51*, 16–24. [CrossRef] [PubMed]
13. Deslandes, A.; Parange, N.; Childs, J.T.; Osborne, B.; Bezak, E. Current Status of Transvaginal Ultrasound Accuracy in the Diagnosis of Deep Infiltrating Endometriosis Before Surgery: A Systematic Review of the Literature. *J. Ultrasound Med.* **2020**. [CrossRef] [PubMed]
14. Guerriero, S.; Ajossa, S. Transvaginal ultrasonography in superficial endometriosis. *Aust. N. Z. J. Obstet. Gynaecol.* **2020**, *60*, E5. [CrossRef] [PubMed]

15. Noventa, M.; Scioscia, M.; Schincariol, M.; Cavallin, F.; Pontrelli, G.; Virgilio, B.; Vitale, S.G.; Laganà, A.S.; Dessole, F.; Cosmi, E.; et al. Imaging Modalities for Diagnosis of Deep Pelvic Endometriosis: Comparison between Trans-Vaginal Sonography, Rectal Endoscopy Sonography and Magnetic Resonance Imaging. A Head-to-Head Meta-Analysis. *Diagnostics* **2019**, *9*, 225. [CrossRef]
16. Guerriero, S.; Saba, L.; Pascual, M.A.; Ajossa, S.; Rodriguez, I.; Mais, V.; Alcazar, J.L. Transvaginal ultrasound vs magnetic resonance imaging for diagnosing deep infiltrating endometriosis: Systematic review and meta-analysis. *Ultrasound Obstet. Gynecol.* **2018**, *51*, 586–595. [CrossRef]
17. Scioscia, M.; Bruni, F.; Ceccaroni, M.; Steinkasserer, M.; Stepniewska, A.; Minelli, L. Distribution of endometriotic lesions in endometriosis stage IV supports the menstrual reflux theory and requires specific preoperative assessment and therapy. *Acta Obstet. Gynecol. Scand.* **2011**, *90*, 136–139. [CrossRef]
18. Chamié, L.P.; Ribeiro, D.M.F.R.; Tiferes, D.A.; de Macedo Neto, A.C.; Serafini, P.C. Atypical Sites of Deeply Infiltrative Endometriosis: Clinical Characteristics and Imaging Findings. *RadioGraphics* **2018**, *38*, 309–328. [CrossRef]
19. Van den Bosch, T.; Dueholm, M.; Leone, F.P.G.; Valentin, L.; Rasmussen, C.K.; Votino, A.; Van Schoubroeck, D.; Landolfo, C.; Installé, A.J.F.; Guerriero, S.; et al. Terms, definitions and measurements to describe sonographic features of myometrium and uterine masses: A consensus opinion from the Morphological Uterus Sonographic Assessment (MUSA) group. *Ultrasound Obstet. Gynecol.* **2015**, *46*, 284–298. [CrossRef]
20. Paul, P.G.; Gulati, G.; Shintre, H.; Mannur, S.; Paul, G.; Mehta, S. Extrauterine adenomyoma: A review of the literature. *Eur. J. Obstet. Gynecol. Reprod. Biol.* **2018**, *228*, 130–136. [CrossRef]
21. Testa, A.C.; Di Legge, A.; Bonatti, M.; Manfredi, R.; Scambia, G. Imaging techniques for evaluation of uterine myomas. *Best Pract. Res. Clin. Obstet. Gynaecol.* **2016**, *34*, 37–53. [CrossRef] [PubMed]
22. Exacoustos, C.; Zupi, E.; Piccione, E. Ultrasound Imaging for Ovarian and Deep Infiltrating Endometriosis. *Semin. Reprod. Med.* **2017**, *35*, 005–024. [CrossRef]
23. Na, K.; Park, S.Y.; Kim, H.-S. Clinicopathological Characteristics of Primary Ovarian Adenomyoma: A Single-institutional Experience. *Anticancer Res.* **2017**, *37*, 2565–2574. [CrossRef] [PubMed]
24. Sokalska, A.; Timmerman, D.; Testa, A.C.; Van Holsbeke, C.; Lissoni, A.A.; Leone, F.P.G.; Jurkovic, D.; Valentin, L. Diagnostic accuracy of transvaginal ultrasound examination for assigning a specific diagnosis to adnexal masses. *Ultrasound Obstet. Gynecol.* **2009**, *34*, 462–470. [CrossRef]
25. Valentin, L. Characterising acute gynaecological pathology with ultrasound: An overview and case examples. *Best Pract. Res. Clin. Obstet. Gynaecol.* **2009**, *23*, 577–593. [CrossRef]
26. Sayasneh, A.; Ekechi, C.; Ferrara, L.; Kaijser, J.; Stalder, C.; Sur, S.; Timmerman, D.; Bourne, T. The characteristic ultrasound features of specific types of ovarian pathology (review). *Int. J. Oncol.* **2015**, *46*, 445–458. [CrossRef]
27. Moro, F.; Zannoni, G.F.; Arciuolo, D.; Pasciuto, T.; Amoroso, S.; Mascilini, F.; Mainenti, S.; Scambia, G.; Testa, A.C. Imaging in gynecological disease (11): Clinical and ultrasound features of mucinous ovarian tumors. *Ultrasound Obstet. Gynecol.* **2017**, *50*, 261–270. [CrossRef]
28. Van Holsbeke, C.; Van Calster, B.; Guerriero, S.; Savelli, L.; Paladini, D.; Lissoni, A.A.; Czekierdowski, A.; Fischerova, D.; Zhang, J.; Mestdagh, G.; et al. Endometriomas: Their ultrasound characteristics. *Ultrasound Obstet. Gynecol.* **2010**, *35*, 730–740. [CrossRef]
29. Timmerman, D.; Valentin, L.; Bourne, T.H.; Collins, W.P.; Verrelst, H.; Vergote, I. International Ovarian Tumor Analysis (IOTA) Group Terms, definitions and measurements to describe the sonographic features of adnexal tumors: A consensus opinion from the International Ovarian Tumor Analysis (IOTA) Group. *Ultrasound Obstet. Gynecol.* **2000**, *16*, 500–505. [CrossRef]
30. Van Holsbeke, C.; Van Calster, B.; Guerriero, S.; Savelli, L.; Leone, F.; Fischerova, D.; Czekierdowski, A.; Fruscio, R.; Veldman, J.; Van de Putte, G.; et al. Imaging in gynecology: How good are we in identifying endometriomas? *Facts Views Vis. ObGyn* **2009**, *1*, 7–17.
31. Timor-Tritsch, I.E.; Lerner, J.P.; Monteagudo, A.; Murphy, K.E.; Heller, D.S. Transvaginal sonographic markers of tubal inflammatory disease. *Ultrasound Obstet. Gynecol.* **1998**, *12*, 56–66. [CrossRef] [PubMed]
32. Van den Bosch, T.; de Bruijn, A.M.; de Leeuw, R.A.; Dueholm, M.; Exacoustos, C.; Valentin, L.; Bourne, T.; Timmerman, D.; Huirne, J.A.F. Sonographic classification and reporting system for diagnosing adenomyosis. *Ultrasound Obstet. Gynecol.* **2019**, *53*, 576–582. [CrossRef] [PubMed]

33. Gründker, C.; Günthert, A.R.; Emons, G. Hormonal heterogeneity of endometrial cancer. *Adv. Exp. Med. Biol.* **2008**, *630*, 166–188. [CrossRef] [PubMed]
34. Yu, O.; Schulze-Rath, R.; Grafton, J.; Hansen, K.; Scholes, D.; Reed, S.D. Adenomyosis incidence, prevalence and treatment: United States population-based study 2006–2015. *Am. J. Obstet. Gynecol.* **2020**, *223*, 94.e1–94.e10. [CrossRef] [PubMed]
35. Chapron, C.; Vannuccini, S.; Santulli, P.; Abrão, M.S.; Carmona, F.; Fraser, I.S.; Gordts, S.; Guo, S.-W.; Just, P.-A.; Noël, J.-C.; et al. Diagnosing adenomyosis: An integrated clinical and imaging approach. *Hum. Reprod. Update* **2020**, *26*, 392–411. [CrossRef]
36. Scioscia, M.; Noventa, M.; Laganà, A.S. Abnormal uterine bleeding and the risk of endometrial cancer: Can subendometrial vascular ultrasound be of help to discriminate cancer from adenomyosis? *Am. J. Obstet. Gynecol.* **2020**, *223*, 605–606. [CrossRef]
37. Guerriero, S.; Ajossa, S.; Gerada, M.; D'Aquila, M.; Piras, B.; Melis, G.B. "Tenderness-guided" transvaginal ultrasonography: A new method for the detection of deep endometriosis in patients with chronic pelvic pain. *Fertil. Steril.* **2007**, *88*, 1293–1297. [CrossRef]
38. Shobeiri, S.A.; Rostaminia, G.; White, D.; Quiroz, L.H.; Nihira, M.A. Evaluation of Vaginal Cysts and Masses by 3-Dimensional Endovaginal and Endoanal Sonography. *J. Ultrasound Med.* **2013**, *32*, 1499–1507. [CrossRef]
39. Testa, A.C.; Ludovisi, M.; Mascilini, F.; Di Legge, A.; Malaggese, M.; Fagotti, A.; Fanfani, F.; Salerno, M.G.; Ercoli, A.; Scambia, G.; et al. Ultrasound evaluation of intra-abdominal sites of disease to predict likelihood of suboptimal cytoreduction in advanced ovarian cancer: A prospective study. *Ultrasound Obstet. Gynecol.* **2012**, *39*, 99–105. [CrossRef]
40. Savelli, L.; Manuzzi, L.; Pollastri, P.; Mabrouk, M.; Seracchioli, R.; Venturoli, S. Diagnostic accuracy and potential limitations of transvaginal sonography for bladder endometriosis. *Ultrasound Obstet. Gynecol.* **2009**, *34*, 595–600. [CrossRef]
41. Chiantera, V.; Petrillo, M.; Abesadze, E.; Sozzi, G.; Dessole, M.; Catello Di Donna, M.; Scambia, G.; Sehouli, J.; Mechsner, S. Laparoscopic Neuronavigation for Deep Lateral Pelvic Endometriosis: Clinical and Surgical Implications. *J. Minim. Invasive Gynecol.* **2018**, *25*, 1217–1223. [CrossRef] [PubMed]
42. Guerriero, S.; Ajossa, S.; Minguez, J.A.; Jurado, M.; Mais, V.; Melis, G.B.; Alcazar, J.L. Accuracy of transvaginal ultrasound for diagnosis of deep endometriosis in uterosacral ligaments, rectovaginal septum, vagina and bladder: Systematic review and meta-analysis. *Ultrasound Obstet. Gynecol.* **2015**, *46*, 534–545. [CrossRef] [PubMed]
43. Mabrouk, M.; Raimondo, D.; Arena, A.; Iodice, R.; Altieri, M.; Sutherland, N.; Salucci, P.; Moro, E.; Seracchioli, R. Parametrial Endometriosis: The Occult Condition that Makes the Hard Harder. *J. Minim. Invasive Gynecol.* **2019**, *26*, 871–876. [CrossRef] [PubMed]
44. Scioscia, M.; Virgilio, B.A.; Scardapane, A.; Pontrelli, G. Fusion Imaging: A Novel Diagnostic Tool for Nerve-sparing Surgery for Deep Infiltrating Endometriosis. *J. Minim. Invasive Gynecol.* **2020**, *27*, 246–247. [CrossRef]
45. Leonardi, M.; Martins, W.P.; Espada, M.; Arianayagam, M.; Condous, G. Proposed technique to visualize and classify uterosacral ligament deep endometriosis with and without infiltration into parametrium or torus uterinus. *Ultrasound Obstet. Gynecol.* **2020**, *55*, 137–139. [CrossRef]
46. Alcazar, J.L.; García, E.; Machuca, M.; Quintana, R.; Escrig, J.; Chacón, E.; Mínguez, J.A.; Chiva, L. Magnetic resonance imaging and ultrasound for assessing parametrial infiltration in cervical cancer. A systematic review and meta-analysis. *Med. Ultrason.* **2020**, *22*, 85–91. [CrossRef]
47. Scioscia, M. Ureteral endometriosis: Correlation between ultrasonography and laparoscopy: Ureteral endometriosis. *Ultrasound Obstet. Gynecol.* **2019**, *53*, 706–708. [CrossRef]
48. Virgilio, B.A.; Pontrelli, G.; Trevisan, P.; Sacchi, D.; Bernardini, T.; Scioscia, M. Incidental diagnosis on transvaginal ultrasound of appendiceal mucocele arising on low-grade appendiceal mucinous neoplasm. *Ultrasound Obstet. Gynecol.* **2019**, *54*, 412–414. [CrossRef]
49. Sima, R.-M.; Radosa, J.C.; Zamfir, R.; Ionescu, C.-A.; Carp, D.; Iordache, I.-I.; Stănescu, A.-D.; Pleş, L. Novel diagnosis of mesenteric endometrioma: Case report. *Medicine (Baltimore)* **2019**, *98*, e16432. [CrossRef]
50. Scioscia, M.; Zanetti, I.; Raspanti, X.; Spoto, E.; Portuese, A.; Noventa, M.; Pontrelli, G.; Greco, P.; Virgilio, B.A. Ultrasound Differential Diagnosis in Deep Infiltrating Endometriosis of the Urinary Tract. *J. Ultrasound Med.* **2020**. [CrossRef]

51. Scardapane, A.; Lorusso, F.; Francavilla, M.; Bettocchi, S.; Fascilla, F.D.; Angelelli, G.; Scioscia, M. Magnetic Resonance Colonography May Predict the Need for Bowel Resection in Colorectal Endometriosis. *BioMed Res. Int.* **2017**, *2017*, 1–7. [CrossRef] [PubMed]
52. Kammann, S.; Menias, C.; Hara, A.; Moshiri, M.; Siegel, C.; Safar, B.; Brandes, S.; Shaaban, A.; Sandrasegaran, K. Genital and reproductive organ complications of Crohn disease: Technical considerations as it relates to perianal disease, imaging features, and implications on management. *Abdom. Radiol.* **2017**, *42*, 1752–1761. [CrossRef] [PubMed]
53. Nezhat, C.; Li, A.; Falik, R.; Copeland, D.; Razavi, G.; Shakib, A.; Mihailide, C.; Bamford, H.; DiFrancesco, L.; Tazuke, S.; et al. Bowel endometriosis: Diagnosis and management. *Am. J. Obstet. Gynecol.* **2018**, *218*, 549–562. [CrossRef] [PubMed]
54. Scioscia, M.; Orlandi, S.; Trivella, G.; Portuese, A.; Bettocchi, S.; Pontrelli, G.; Bocus, P.; Anna Virgilio, B. Sonographic Differential Diagnosis in Deep Infiltrating Endometriosis: The Bowel. *BioMed Res. Int.* **2019**, *2019*, 1–9. [CrossRef] [PubMed]
55. Fujita, M.; Manabe, N.; Honda, K.; Murao, T.; Osawa, M.; Kawai, R.; Akiyama, T.; Shiotani, A.; Haruma, K.; Hata, J. Usefulness of Ultrasonography for Diagnosis of Small Bowel Tumors: A Comparison Between Ultrasonography and Endoscopic Modalities. *Medicine* **2015**, *94*, e1464. [CrossRef] [PubMed]
56. Kołodziej, A.; Krajewski, W.; Dołowy, Ł.; Hirnle, L. Urinary Tract Endometriosis. *Urol. J.* **2015**, *12*, 2213–2217.
57. Pateman, K.; Holland, T.K.; Knez, J.; Derdelis, G.; Cutner, A.; Saridogan, E.; Jurkovic, D. Should a detailed ultrasound examination of the complete urinary tract be routinely performed in women with suspected pelvic endometriosis? *Hum. Reprod.* **2015**, *30*, 2802–2807. [CrossRef]
58. Testa, A.C.; Di Legge, A.; De Blasis, I.; Cristina Moruzzi, M.; Bonatti, M.; Collarino, A.; Rufini, V.; Manfredi, R. Imaging techniques for the evaluation of cervical cancer. *Best Pract. Res. Clin. Obstet. Gynaecol.* **2014**, *28*, 741–768. [CrossRef] [PubMed]
59. Smereczyński, A.; Szopiński, T.; Gołąbek, T.; Ostasz, O.; Bojko, S. Sonography of tumors and tumor-like lesions that mimic carcinoma of the urinary bladder. *J. Ultrason.* **2014**, *14*, 36–48. [CrossRef]
60. Pavlica, P.; Gaudiano, C.; Barozzi, L. Sonography of the bladder. *World J. Urol.* **2004**, *22*, 328–334. [CrossRef]
61. Barra, F.; Scala, C.; Biscaldi, E.; Vellone, V.G.; Ceccaroni, M.; Terrone, C.; Ferrero, S. Ureteral endometriosis: A systematic review of epidemiology, pathogenesis, diagnosis, treatment, risk of malignant transformation and fertility. *Hum. Reprod. Update* **2018**, *24*, 710–730. [CrossRef] [PubMed]
62. Guerriero, S.; Conway, F.; Pascual, M.A.; Graupera, B.; Ajossa, S.; Neri, M.; Musa, E.; Pedrassani, M.; Alcazar, J.L. Ultrasonography and Atypical Sites of Endometriosis. *Diagnostics (Basel)* **2020**, *10*, 345. [CrossRef] [PubMed]
63. Mascilini, F.; Moruzzi, C.; Giansiracusa, C.; Guastafierro, F.; Savelli, L.; De Meis, L.; Epstein, E.; Timor-Tritsch, I.E.; Mailath-Pokorny, M.; Ercoli, A.; et al. Imaging in gynecological disease. 10: Clinical and ultrasound characteristics of decidualized endometriomas surgically removed during pregnancy. *Ultrasound Obstet. Gynecol.* **2014**, *44*, 354–360. [CrossRef] [PubMed]
64. Noventa, M.; Saccardi, C.; Litta, P.; Vitagliano, A.; D'Antona, D.; Abdulrahim, B.; Duncan, A.; Alexander-Sefre, F.; Aldrich, C.J.; Quaranta, M.; et al. Ultrasound techniques in the diagnosis of deep pelvic endometriosis: Algorithm based on a systematic review and meta-analysis. *Fertil. Steril.* **2015**, *104*, 366–383.e2. [CrossRef] [PubMed]
65. Grigore, M.; Socolov, D.; Pavaleanu, I.; Scripcariu, I.; Grigore, A.M.; Micu, R. Abdominal wall endometriosis: An update in clinical, imagistic features, and management options. *Med. Ultrason.* **2017**, *19*, 430. [CrossRef]
66. Morales Martínez, C.; Tejuca Somoano, S. Abdominal wall endometriosis. *Am. J. Obstet. Gynecol.* **2017**, *217*, 701–702. [CrossRef]
67. Ecker, A.M.; Donnellan, N.M.; Shepherd, J.P.; Lee, T.T.M. Abdominal wall endometriosis: 12 years of experience at a large academic institution. *Am. J. Obstet. Gynecol.* **2014**, *211*, 363.e1–363.e5. [CrossRef]
68. Bean, E.; Chaggar, P.; Thanatsis, N.; Dooley, W.; Bottomley, C.; Jurkovic, D. Intra- and interobserver reproducibility of pelvic ultrasound for the detection and measurement of endometriotic lesions. *Hum. Reprod. Open* **2020**, *2020*, hoaa001. [CrossRef]

69. Guerriero, S.; Pascual, M.A.; Ajossa, S.; Rodriguez, I.; Zajicek, M.; Rolla, M.; Rams Llop, N.; Yulzari, V.; Bardin, R.; Buonomo, F.; et al. Learning curve for ultrasonographic diagnosis of deep infiltrating endometriosis using structured offline training program. *Ultrasound Obstet. Gynecol.* **2019**, *54*, 262–269. [CrossRef]
70. Eisenberg, V.H.; Alcazar, J.L.; Arbib, N.; Schiff, E.; Achiron, R.; Goldenberg, M.; Soriano, D. Applying a statistical method in transvaginal ultrasound training: Lessons from the learning curve cumulative summation test (LC-CUSUM) for endometriosis mapping. *Gynecol. Surg.* **2017**, *14*, 19. [CrossRef]

Publisher's Note: MDPI stays neutral with regard to jurisdictional claims in published maps and institutional affiliations.

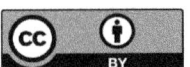

© 2020 by the authors. Licensee MDPI, Basel, Switzerland. This article is an open access article distributed under the terms and conditions of the Creative Commons Attribution (CC BY) license (http://creativecommons.org/licenses/by/4.0/).

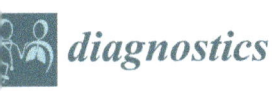

Comment

Transvaginal Strain Elastosonography May Help in the Differential Diagnosis of Endometriosis?

Gábor Szabó [1,*], István Madár [1], Attila Bokor [1] and János Rigó, Jr. [1,2]

1. Department of Obstetrics and Gynecology, Faculty of Medicine, Semmelweis University, Baross utca 27, 1088 Budapest, Hungary; madar.istvan@med.semmelweis-univ.hu (I.M.); bokor.attila@med.semmelweis-univ.hu (A.B.); rigo.janos@med.semmelweis-univ.hu (J.R.J.)
2. Department of Clinical Studies in Obstetrics and Gynecology, Faculty of Health Sciences, Semmelweis University, Vas utca 17, 1088 Budapest, Hungary
* Correspondence: szabo.gabor6@med.semmelweis-univ.hu; Tel.: +36-20-455-4710

Dear Editor,

We read with great interest the paper entitled "Differential Diagnosis of Endometriosis by Ultrasound: A Rising Challenge" of Scioscia et al. [1]. We fully agree with the authors that with the spread of the International Deep Endometriosis Analysis (IDEA) group protocol, the detection rate of endometriosis has significantly increased among users. As the number of detected cases increases, so does the number of false positive results. Because of the heterogeneous, multiform and often non-specific symptoms of endometriosis, differential diagnostic is a real challenge. The authors' excellent article provides a comprehensive review of the possible involved organs.

They correctly pointed out that deep endometriosis infiltrates the anterior wall of the rectum. Endometriotic nodules affecting the rectum and rectosigmoid bowel are hypo- or anechogenic. Due to scarring, they show with color Doppler only a minimal signalling. We have previously reported that infiltrating lesions of rectal endometriosis appear to be stiffer than sections of healthy intestinal wall by transvaginal strain elastosonographic examination [2] (Figure 1A). A strain ratio (SR) of 2.0 serves as a cut-off value for the optimal distinction.

However, stenosis of the rectosigmoid bowel is not only caused by endometriosis. Colorectal cancer has the highest incidence rates of all gastrointestinal malignancies worldwide and also leads to changes in the ultrasound image of the bowel [3]. Rectal cancer usually grows outward and it can reach the serosa, contrary to deep infiltrating endometriosis lesions infiltrating inward. With a color Doppler ultrasound examination, rectal cancer shows increased vascularity [4]. Previously with transrectal elastosonographic examination, benign adenomas did not show a significant difference compared to a healthy intestinal wall ($SR \leq 1.25$). Malignant tumors have an $SR > 1.25$ [5]. Stiffness of early rectal cancer—T1 and T2 stages according to the TNM classification of malignant tumors—in contrast to deep endometriosis, is no more than twice that of a healthy, intact bowel wall [6]. There is a tendency for a higher fibrosis score ($SR > 2.0$) only for tumors staged as T3 or T4. This observation may provide additional information for differential diagnosis. In our practice, a 37-year-old patient with suspicious signs for deep endometriosis (infertility, diarrhoea and bloating) was examined with transvaginal sonography. On the anterior wall of the rectum, a stenosing lesion of 2 cm in diameter was visible at a 15 cm distance from the anal verge. Color Doppler showed intense vascularisation. The layers of muscularis propria and subserosa seemed to be intact. With strain elastography, the serosa was without interruption. The strain ratio between lesion and normal bowel wall was 1.33 (Figure 1B). Histological examination confirmed well-differentiated adenocarcinoma from the sample, obtained during the performed colonoscopy.

Inflammatory bowel diseases (IBDs) are like endometriosis, also being common pathologic conditions of unknown origin. Epidemiological studies reported a positive association between endometriosis and IBD [7]. Crohn's disease occurs predominantly in young women in their peak reproductive years. Inflammation of the intestinal wall can lead to adhesions, perforations and fistula formation. Later, it can also cause fibrosis in the bowel wall. No correlation was previously observed between mean strain ratio and fibrosis score [8]. In Crohn's disease, similar to endometriosis, patients may develop symptoms like bloating, haematochezia and diarrhoea. In our practice, a 35-year-old patient with such complaints was diagnosed with deep infiltrating endometriosis in the rectovaginal space with palpation. Colonoscopic examination showed protrusion in the lumen of the rectum at a 15 cm distance from the anal verge. Transvaginal strain sonoelastography showed a stiff nodule of 3 cm in diameter. In the same patient, transvaginal ultrasound also revealed, on the right side, adhesions between the small intestine and thickening of the intestinal wall. A conventional ultrasound image of the intestinal conglomerate was similar to multicentric deep endometriosis in the bowel, but the elastostonography did not confirm this. Elastosonographic examination could not isolate a stiff nodule corresponding to deep endometriosis. Instead, a pattern suggestive of diffuse fibrosis appeared (Figure 1C). During surgery in the rectovaginal space, we excised a deep endometriosis nodule of 3 cm in diameter. Histological examination verified endometriosis. In the ileocoecal region, intraoperative peritoneal adhesions and bowel strictures were found resembling endometriosis, but histology confirmed Crohn's disease only.

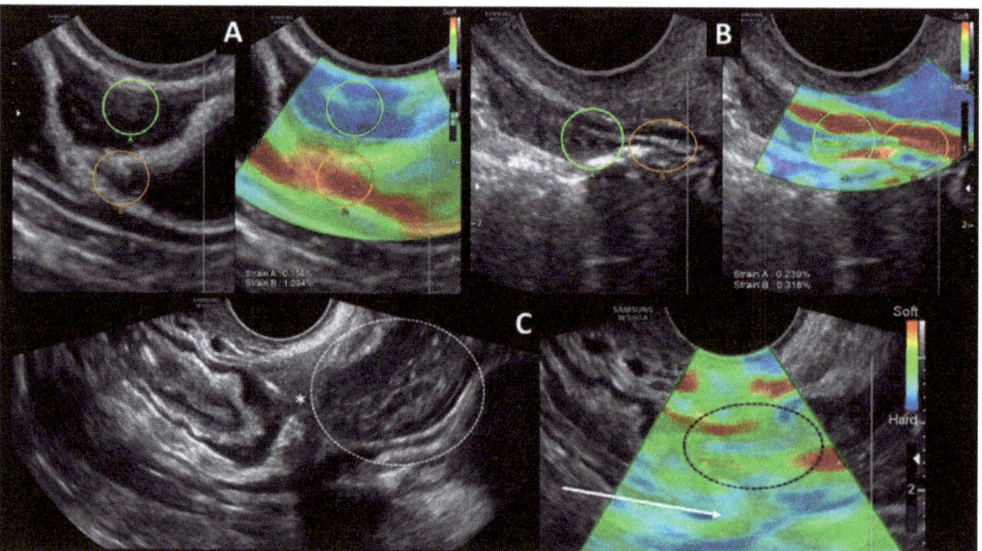

Figure 1. Transvaginal strain elastosonography in different intestinal diseases. Dual-mode greyscale sonographic (left) and strain elastosonography (right) images. (**A**) Deep infiltrating endometriosis on the anterior wall of the rectum. A stiff delineated lesion (blue area) infiltrates through the serosa into the muscularis propria layer. The posterior regular rectal wall is soft (red area). Strain measurement between the lesion in the anterior rectal wall (green circle) and the regular posterior rectal wall (orange circle). The calculated strain ratio (SR) is 7.1. (**B**) Adenocarcinoma on the anterior wall of the rectum. The sonoelastographic appearance of the tumor shows increased stiffness (blue and green area). The serosa of the rectum is uninterrupted (red area). Strain measurement between the tumor (green circle) and the regular rectal wall (orange circle). The calculated strain ratio (SR) is 1.33. (**C**) Sagittal transvaginal sonogram in Crohn's disease. On the greyscale sonographic image (left), thickened intestinal wall (circle) and stricture (asterisk) are visible in the ileocecal region. The sonoelastographic appearance (right) of the intestinal loops does not show a delineated nodule in the area of the stricture (black circle) but diffuse fibrosis between the adhering intestinal loops (arrow).

This is the first case, to the best of our knowledge, in the literature where preoperative differential diagnosis has been achieved with the use of elastosonography by the simultaneous occurrence of deep endometriosis affecting the gastrointestinal tract and Crohn's disease.

As Scioscia et al. conceive in their article, "accurate diagnosis of endometriosis has significant clinical impact and is important for appropriate treatment". To achieve this, an interdisciplinary approach and the appropriate application of different imaging methods are necessary. Transvaginal ultrasound is a widely available, non-invasive technique. In our opinion, sonoelastography can provide additional data as a valuable element of the diagnostic process. It is important for the physician performing the sonography to receive feedback from the surgeon or even be present at the surgery.

Author Contributions: Conceptualisation, G.S. and I.M.; data curation, A.B.; writing—original draft preparation, G.S.; writing—review and editing, G.S. and I.M.; supervision, J.R.J. All authors have read and agreed to the published version of the manuscript.

Funding: This research received no external funding.

Institutional Review Board Statement: The study was conducted according to the guidelines of the Declaration of Helsinki, and approved by the Ethics Committee of OGYÉI/65175/2020, Approval Date: 3 December 2020.

Informed Consent Statement: Informed consent was obtained from all subjects involved in the study.

Data Availability Statement: No new data were created or analyzed in this study. Data sharing is not applicable to this article.

Conflicts of Interest: The authors declare no conflict of interest.

References

Scioscia, M.; Virgilio, B.A.; Laganà, A.S.; Bernardini, T.; Fattizzi, N.; Neri, M.; Guerriero, S. Differential Diagnosis of Endometriosis by Ultrasound: A Rising Challenge. *Diagnostics* **2020**, *10*, 848. [CrossRef] [PubMed]

Szabó, G.; Madár, I.; Bokor, A.; Brubel, R.; Csibi, N.; Rigó, J., Jr. Preoperative mapping of deep infiltrating endometriosis in the posterior compartment using transvaginal strain elastography and IDEA classification. *Ultrasound Obst. Gyn.* **2019**, *54* (Suppl. 1), 50. [CrossRef]

Scioscia, M.; Orlandi, S.; Trivella, G.; Portuese, A.; Bettocchi, S.; Pontrelli, G.; Bocus, P.; Anna Virgilio, B. Sonographic Differential Diagnosis in Deep Infiltrating Endometriosis: The Bowel. *BioMed Res. Int.* **2019**, *2019*, 5958402. [CrossRef] [PubMed]

Sudakoff, G.S.; Quiroz, F.; Foley, W.D. Sonography of anorectal, rectal, and perirectal abnormalities. *Am. J. Roentgenol.* **2002**, *179*, 131–136. [CrossRef] [PubMed]

Bor, R.; Fábián, A.; Szepes, Z. Role of ultrasound in colorectal diseases. *World J. Gastroenterol.* **2016**, *22*, 9477–9487. [CrossRef] [PubMed]

Havre, R.F.; Leh, S.; Gilja, O.H.; Ødegaard, S.; Waage, J.E.; Baatrup, G.; Nesje, L.B. Strain Assessment in Surgically Resected Inflammatory and Neoplastic Bowel Lesions. *Ultraschall Med.* **2014**, *35*, 149–158. [CrossRef] [PubMed]

Chiaffarino, F.; Cipriani, S.; Ricci, E.; Roncella, E.; Mauri, P.A.; Parazzini, F.; Vercellini, P. Endometriosis and inflammatory bowel disease: A systematic review of the literature. *Eur. J. Obstet. Gynecol. Reprod. Biol.* **2020**, *252*, 246–251. [CrossRef] [PubMed]

Serra, C.; Rizzello, F.; Pratico, C.; Felicani, C.; Fiorini, E.; Brugnera, R.; Mazzotta, E.; Giunchi, F.; Fiorentino, M.; D'Errico, A.; et al. Real-time elastography for the detection of fibrotic and inflammatory tissue in patients with stricturing Crohn's disease. *J. Ultrasound* **2017**, *26*, 273–284. [CrossRef] [PubMed]

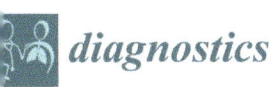

Reply

Transvaginal Strain Elastosonography in the Differential Diagnosis of Rectal Endometriosis: Some Potentials and Limits

Marco Scioscia [1,2,*], Antonio Simone Laganà [3], Giuseppe Caringella [2] and Stefano Guerriero [4,5]

1. Unit of Gynecological Surgery, Mater Dei Hospital, 70125 Bari, BA, Italy
2. Obstetrics and Gynecology, Mater Dei Hospital, 70125 Bari, BA, Italy; caringellagiuseppe@libero.it
3. Department of Obstetrics and Gynecology, "Filippo Del Ponte" Hospital, University of Insubria, 21100 Varese, VA, Italy; antoniosimone.lagana@uninsubria.it
4. Obstetrics and Gynecology, University of Cagliari, 09124 Cagliari, CA, Italy; gineca.sguerriero@tiscali.it
5. Department of Obstetrics and Gynecology, Azienda Ospedaliero Universitaria, Policlinico Universitario Duilio Casula, 09045 Monserrato, CA, Italy
* Correspondence: marcoscioscia@gmail.com

Dear Editor,

We sincerely thank Szabó et al. [1] for their comments on our article [2] and their proposal for improving the differential diagnosis of bowel endometriosis by transvaginal elastosonography (ESG). This technique provides noninvasive information on the elasticity and stiffness of a lesion, as it is based on the principle that the compression of soft tissues produces a greater strain in soft and elastic lesions than in harder, more rigid lesions. The results (calculated strain ratio) depend on the amount of the fibrotic component of the lesion and the surrounding tissue.

Fibrosis is a local reactive response to tissue growth in both endometriosis [3] and cancer [4] while it is secondary to inflammation in inflammatory bowel diseases (IBD) (i.e., Chron's disease) [5]. A correct diagnosis is of key importance, as treatment varies from the need for bowel segmental resection in case of cancer, to possible bowel surgery in endometriosis cases, to medical anti-inflammatory treatment and endoscopic balloon dilation in IBD. As we discussed in a previous article of ours [6], colon cancer growths typically extend outward from the mucosa and reach the serosa, whereas endometriosis lesions grow inward starting from the serosa, so the differential diagnosis is usually not difficult [2]. Patients with IBD commonly develop bowel strictures that may resemble deep infiltrating endometriosis of the bowel at ultrasound.

We agree with Szabó et al. [1] that ESG examination may be of help in the differential diagnosis, as a stiff nodule is not found in IBD. Nevertheless, some aspects related to the technique and diseases should be considered. The strain measurements may show an increased interobserver variability due to the force applied during the transvaginal elastography, even though modern specific ultrasound software provides some information about the pressure made with the probe. The distance between the probe and the lesion represents another limitation, as satisfactory images are more easily acquired if the lesion is relatively close to the probe [7–9]. Morphologic and elastographic scores may differ significantly when the bowel lesion is farther away, such as seen in sigmoid endometriosis (Figure 1B,C). Certainly, the majority of endometriosis lesions of the bowel involve the rectum and the rectosigmoid junction [10] or they are quite proximal to the posterior vaginal fornix where the probe is inserted (Figure 1A). Another aspect that should be considered is the case of large nodules that involve the rectum for more than 5 cm (Figure 1D). ESG is based on differences in stiffness induced by the pathological lesion and the normal adjacent tissue that, in cases of large nodules, may be farther away from the probe, so measurements may be less accurate. Similarly, the reactive fibrosis may present as long tails before and after the nodule that may make it difficult to acquire the reference (normal tissue) for stiffness calculation too far away from the probe (Figure 1E,F).

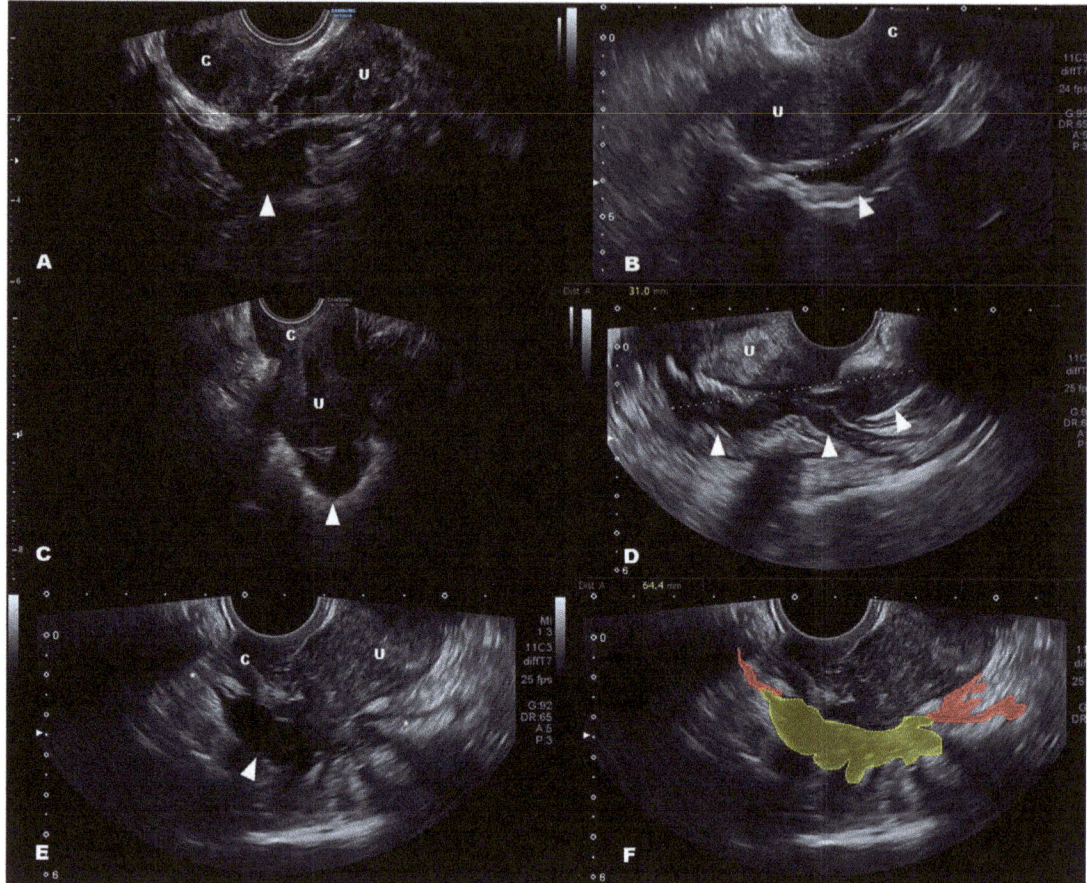

Figure 1. Deep infiltrating endometriosis of the colorectum. (**A,B**) show, respectively, typical nodules (arrow) of the medial and the proximal part of the rectum. (**C**) shows an endometriosis nodule of the sigmoid colon. (**D**) shows a large nodule that involves the rectum, from proximal to distal, and the distal sigmoid. (**E**) shows a nodule that involves the medial and proximal part of the rectum (arrow) with long fibrotic tails (*); (**F**) is explains (**E**) where the nodule is in yellow and the fibrotic tails are in red. Abbreviations: U uterus; C cervix.

In view of this, further studies are required to assess the potential of ESG in improving the detection rate, potential for differential diagnosis, and intra- and inter-observer reproducibility coefficients of this technique.

Author Contributions: Conceptualization, M.S. and S.G.; data curation, M.S., G.C., and A.S.L.; writing—original draft preparation, M.S.; writing—review and editing, A.S.L. and G.C.; supervision S.G. All authors have read and agreed to the published version of the manuscript.

Funding: This research received no external funding.

Institutional Review Board Statement: Not applicable.

Informed Consent Statement: Not applicable.

Data Availability Statement: Not applicable.

Conflicts of Interest: The authors declare no conflict of interest.

References

1. Szabò, G.; Madàr, I.; Bokor, A.; Rigò, J.J. Transvaginal strain elastosonography may help in the differential diagnosis of endometriosis? *Diagnostics* **2020**, *11*, 100. [CrossRef]
2. Scioscia, M.; Virgilio, B.A.; Laganà, A.S.; Bernardini, T.; Fattizzi, N.; Neri, M.; Guerriero, S. Differential Diagnosis of Endometriosis by Ultrasound: A Rising Challenge. *Diagnostics* **2020**, *10*, 848. [CrossRef]
3. Viganò, P.; Ottolina, J.; Bartiromo, L.; Bonavina, G.; Schimberni, M.; Villanacci, R.; Candiani, M. Cellular Components Contributing to Fibrosis in Endometriosis: A Literature Review. *J. Minim. Invasive Gynecol.* **2020**, *27*, 287–295. [CrossRef]
4. Shin, N.; Son, G.M.; Shin, D.-H.; Kwon, M.-S.; Park, B.-S.; Kim, H.-S.; Ryu, D.; Kang, C.-D. Cancer-Associated Fibroblasts and Desmoplastic Reactions Related to Cancer Invasiveness in Patients With Colorectal Cancer. *Ann. Coloproctol.* **2019**, *35*, 36–46. [CrossRef] [PubMed]
5. Bettenworth, D.; Bokemeyer, A.; Baker, M.; Mao, R.; Parker, C.E.; Nguyen, T.; Ma, C.; Panés, J.; Rimola, J.; Fletcher, J.G.; et al. Assessment of Crohn's disease-associated small bowel strictures and fibrosis on cross-sectional imaging: A systematic review. *Gut* **2019**, *68*, 1115–1126. [CrossRef] [PubMed]
6. Scioscia, M.; Orlandi, S.; Trivella, G.; Portuese, A.; Bettocchi, S.; Pontrelli, G.; Bocus, P.; Anna Virgilio, B. Sonographic Differential Diagnosis in Deep Infiltrating Endometriosis: The Bowel. *BioMed Res. Int.* **2019**, *2019*, 5958402. [CrossRef] [PubMed]
7. Hwang, J.A.; Jeong, W.K.; Song, K.D.; Kang, K.A.; Lim, H.K. 2-D Shear Wave Elastography for Focal Lesions in Liver Phantoms: Effects of Background Stiffness, Depth and Size of Focal Lesions on Stiffness Measurement. *Ultrasound Med. Biol.* **2019**, *45*, 3261–3268. [CrossRef] [PubMed]
8. Song, G.; Jing, L.; Yan, M.; Cong, S.; Xuejiao, W. Influence of various breast factors on the quality of strain elastograms. *J. Ultrasound Med.* **2015**, *34*, 395–400. [CrossRef]
9. Park, H.S.; Kim, Y.J.; Yu, M.H.; Jung, S.I.; Jeon, H.J. Shear Wave Elastography of Focal Liver Lesion: Intraobserver Reproducibility and Elasticity Characterization. *Ultrasound Q.* **2015**, *31*, 262–271. [CrossRef]
10. Scioscia, M.; Bruni, F.; Ceccaroni, M.; Steinkasserer, M.; Stepniewska, A.; Minelli, L. Distribution of endometriotic lesions in endometriosis stage IV supports the menstrual reflux theory and requires specific preoperative assessment and therapy. *Acta Obstet. Gynecol. Scand.* **2011**, *90*, 136–139. [CrossRef] [PubMed]

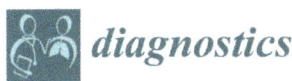

Article

A Prospective Study Comparing Three-Dimensional Rectal Water Contrast Transvaginal Ultrasonography and Computed Tomographic Colonography in the Diagnosis of Rectosigmoid Endometriosis

Fabio Barra [1,2], Ennio Biscaldi [3], Carolina Scala [4], Antonio Simone Laganà [5], Valerio Gaetano Vellone [6], Cesare Stabilini [6], Fabio Ghezzi [5] and Simone Ferrero [1,2,*]

1. Academic Unit of Obstetrics and Gynecology, IRCCS Ospedale Policlinico San Martino, 16132 Genoa, Italy; fabio.barra@icloud.com
2. Department of Neurosciences, Rehabilitation, Ophthalmology, Genetics, Maternal and Child Health (DiNOGMI), University of Genoa, 16132 Genoa, Italy
3. Department of Radiology, Galliera Hospital, 16142, Genoa, Italy; ennio.biscaldi@gmail.com
4. Unit of Obstetrics and Gynecology, Gaslini Institute, 16147 Genova, Italy; carolinascala@icloud.com
5. Department of Obstetrics and Gynecology, "Filippo Del Ponte" Hospital, University of Insubria, 21100 Varese, Italy; antoniosimone.lagana@uninsubria.it (A.S.L.); fabio.ghezzi@uninsubria.it (F.G.)
6. Department of Surgical and Diagnostic Sciences, IRCCS Ospedale Policlinico San Martino, 16132 Genoa, Italy; vgvellone@gmail.com (V.G.V.); cesare.stabilini@unige.it (C.S.)
* Correspondence: simoneferrero@me.com; Tel.: +39-34-7721-1682

Received: 31 March 2020; Accepted: 23 April 2020; Published: 24 April 2020

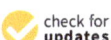

Abstract: (1) Objectives: In patients with symptoms suggestive of rectosigmoid endometriosis, imaging techniques are required to confirm the presence and establish the extent of the disease. The objective of the current study was to compare the performance of three-dimensional rectal water contrast transvaginal ultrasonography (3D-RWC-TVS) and computed tomographic colonography (CTC) in predicting the presence and characteristics of rectosigmoid endometriosis. (2) Methods: This prospective study included patients with suspicion of rectosigmoid endometriosis who underwent both 3D-RWC-TVS and CTC and subsequently were surgically treated. The findings of imaging techniques were compared with surgical and histological results. (3) Results: Out of 68 women included in the study, 37 (48.9; 95% C.I. 38.2–59.7%) had rectosigmoid nodules and underwent bowel surgery. There was no significant difference in the accuracy of 3D-RWC-TVS and CTC in diagnosing the presence of rectosigmoid endometriotic nodules ($p = 0.118$), although CTC was more precise in diagnosing endometriosis located in the sigmoid ($p = 0.016$). 3D-RWC-TVS and CTC had similar precision in estimating the largest diameter of the main endometriotic nodule ($p = 0.099$) and, in patients undergoing segmental resection, the degree of the stenosis of the bowel lumen ($p = 0.293$). CTC was more accurate in estimating the distance between the lower margin of the intestinal nodule and the anal verge ($p = 0.030$) but was less tolerated than 3D-RWC-TVS ($p < 0.001$). (4) Conclusion: This was the first study comparing the performance of 3D-RWC-TVS and CTC in the diagnosis of rectosigmoid endometriosis. Both techniques allowed for the evaluation of the profile of the bowel lumen in a pseudoendoscopic fashion and had a similar performance for the diagnosis of rectosigmoid endometriosis, although CTC was more accurate in diagnosing and characterizing sigmoid nodules.

Keywords: rectosigmoid endometriosis; three-dimensional rectal water contrast transvaginal ultrasonography; computed colonography; bowel stenosis; bowel endometriosis; intestinal segmental resection

1. Introduction

Rectosigmoid endometriosis is one of the most severe forms of endometriosis, and it is defined by the presence of endometriotic glands and stroma infiltrating at least the muscularis propria of the rectosigmoid colon. Besides pain symptoms, this disease may cause several intestinal complaints that often worsen during the menstrual cycle (such as painful bowel movements, abdominal bloating, cyclical diarrhea or constipation, passage of mucus with the stools and rectal bleeding) [1]. An accurate preoperative diagnostic workup of rectosigmoid endometriosis is necessary to provide the patient with informed consent on the benefits and risks of the potential treatments (hormonal therapies or surgical approach) and to obtain adequate informed consent in case of surgery [2,3]. Furthermore, knowing the presence of bowel endometriosis preoperatively allows planning surgery with an appropriate multidisciplinary team, including the colorectal surgeon. Finally, the features of intestinal nodules may be relevant for some surgeons to choose the technique used to excise rectosigmoid nodules (shaving, discoid excision, or segmental bowel resection) [4,5].

Several ultrasonographic and radiological techniques (such as transvaginal ultrasonography (TVS), magnetic resonance imaging (MR), and rectal endoscopic ultrasonography) have been used for diagnosing rectosigmoid endometriosis [6]. In most of these techniques, the intestinal lumen is not distended, and, therefore, it is not possible to reliably estimate the degrees of stenosis caused by rectosigmoid nodules. This parameter is relevant for patients undergoing surgery, as it may affect the surgical technique. In addition, the degree of stenosis of the intestinal lumen is important for patients undergoing hormonal therapies in order to predict the risk of stenosis and occlusive symptoms during treatment. Finally, this parameter is relevant for patients desiring to conceive to minimize the risk of intestinal occlusion during pregnancy [7–11].

TVS is the first-line imaging technique in patients with suspicion of rectosigmoid endometriosis and, when performed by expert ultrasonographers in referral centers specializing in the diagnosis of endometriosis, it may provide most of the information useful to the clinicians [6]. Over the last ten years, several ultrasonographic techniques based on the distention of the vagina and/or rectosigmoid with saline solution and/or ultrasonographic gel have been proposed with the aim of improving the diagnosis of deep infiltrating endometriosis [12]. Among the others, rectal water contrast transvaginal ultrasonography (RWC-TVS) has been employed in this setting, demonstrating a high accuracy in ruling out the presence of rectosigmoid endometriosis [13–15].

Three-dimensional (3D) reconstructions convert standard 2D grayscale acquisitions into a volumetric dataset. 3D ultrasound has been employed for the evaluation of many gynecological diseases, including uterine shape abnormalities (e.g., Mullerian duct abnormalities), uterine intracavitary pathology (submucous uterine fibroids or endometrial polyps) [16]. The use of 3D-TVS has also been proposed for the diagnosis of deep endometriosis [17–19].

In general, radiological techniques can be used to establish the presence and extent of rectosigmoid endometriosis, particularly when there is suspicion of disease despite negative ultrasonographic findings and/or of the presence of multifocal disease with sigmoid or upper intestinal nodules. Moreover, in order to plan surgery, nowadays the role of radiologic imaging still remains relevant and many patients with clinical suspicion of rectosigmoid endometriosis are routinely referred to radiologists for the diagnosis of intestinal endometriosis [20,21].

Computed colonography (CTC) is used worldwide for the screening of colorectal cancer. Over the last ten years, several studies showed that CTC has high diagnostic performance in the diagnosis of rectosigmoid endometriosis [22–26]; this exam is as accurate as TVS in diagnosing rectosigmoid endometriosis and has the advantage of investigating the whole colon [27]. Image post-processing is performed using workstations suitable for 3D data management and reconstruction. The evaluation of CTC also includes the anatomic reconstruction by 3D images; in case of large bowel evaluation, 3D review typically refers to an optical colonoscopy-like endoluminal fly-through (FT) of a 3D reconstructed colon.

At the best of our knowledge, no previous study has compared the diagnostic performance of 3D-rectal water contrast transvaginal ultrasonography (3D-RWC-TVS) and CTC in the diagnosis of rectosigmoid endometriosis. As both techniques are based on the distention of the rectosigmoid and allow the evaluation of the profile of the bowel lumen in a pseudoendoscopic fashion, the objective of the current study was to compare the diagnostic performance of 3D-RWC-TVS and CTC in predicting the presence and characteristics of rectosigmoid endometriosis.

2. Materials and Methods

The primary objective of the study was to compare the performance of 3D-RWC-TVS and CTC in the diagnosis of rectosigmoid endometriosis. The secondary objectives were to compare the precision of the two techniques in estimating the length (mid-sagittal diameter) of the intestinal nodules, the presence of multifocal disease (presence of one or more lesions affecting the sigmoid colon that are associated with a colorectal primary lesion) and the distance between the lower margin of the nodules and the anal verge.

This was a prospective study performed between March 2017 and September 2019. Subjects of the study were recruited among patients referred to our institution because of pain and intestinal symptoms suggestive of rectosigmoid endometriosis. Some patients had histological diagnosis of pelvic endometriosis during previous surgery. Previous surgical diagnosis of intestinal endometriosis, previous radiological diagnosis of intestinal endometriosis (based on MR or double-contrast barium enema), history of colorectal surgery (except appendectomy), contraindications to bowel preparation or CTC (such as non-compliant patients), previous bilateral ovariectomy, or psychiatric disorders were exclusion criteria for this study.

Study patients underwent 3D-RWC-TVS performed by an ultrasonographer highly skilled in the diagnosis of deep endometriosis. CTC was done within the following three months by a radiologist expert in the diagnosis of deep endometriosis, blinded to the results of the previous ultrasonographic exam.

As described in the consensus opinion from the International Deep Endometriosis Analysis (IDEA) group, intestinal nodules located below the level of the insertion of the uterosacral ligaments on the cervix were defined as "anterior lower rectal nodules", those above this level were defined as "anterior upper rectal nodules", those at the level of the uterine fundus were defined as "rectosigmoid junction nodules" and those above the level of the uterine fundus were defined as "anterior sigmoid nodules" [6]. Bowel stenosis was defined as a reduction in lumen, by measuring the smallest stricture diameter and comparing it with the closest healthy bowel lumen diameter.

Patients underwent surgery within six months from the performance of 3D-RWC-TVS. The results of CTC and 3D-RWC-TVS were compared with surgical and histological findings.

The local ethics committee approved the study protocol (CE2439PRNO161219-24/2020). Patients participating in the study provided written informed consent. This study was registered in Clinicaltrial.gov (NCT04295343).

2.1. Three-Dimensional Rectal Water Contrast Transvaginal Sonography

A sonographer (S.F.) with extensive experience in the diagnosis of intestinal endometriosis (>500 exams every year) performed all the exams. 3D-RWC-TVS was performed by Voluson E6 and E10 machines equipped with transvaginal transducers (GE Healthcare Ultrasound, Milwaukee, WI, USA). Patients received a rectal enema (133 mL of monobasic sodium phosphate anhydrous; Clisma Lax; Sofar, Milan, Italy) a few hours before TVS. A total of 300–400 mL of saline solution was employed to distend the rectosigmoid under ultrasonographic control, by using a catheter connected to a 100 mL syringe introduced in the anus [14,28].

During the ultrasonographic scan, acquisitions of images by 3D rendering were made in the sagittal and coronal planes. Two specific quality enhancement tools (GE Healthcare Ultrasound, Milwaukee, WI, USA) were applied during 3D rendering: advanced Speckle Reduction Imaging (SRI), which helps heighten the visibility of lesions with high-definition contrast resolution and CrossXBeamCRI[TM], which improves the enhancement of tissue and border differentiation. On the 3D rendering, rectosigmoid lesions typically appear as spiculated lesions with a retracting line all around the nodule (Figure 1) [18].

Multiple acquisitions were performed to characterize the endometriotic nodules, in particular, measuring their largest diameter and their distance from the anal verge. When the volume acquisition was completed, the data file was sent via Digital Imaging and Communication in Medicine (DICOM) to a personal computer and stored in order to be analysed by the use of an appropriate software (4Dview 5.0; GE Healthcare Ultrasound, Milwaukee, WI, USA). All the acquisitions were examined by another sonographer who has performed over 1000 analysis of 3D imaging related to deep endometriosis in his life (F.B.). This sonographer was blinded to the results of the 2D-RWC-TVS. For estimating the stenosis, at least three measurements of the diameter of rectosigmoid lumen were performed above and below the nodule (mean of all measurements) in a healthy bowel; close to the nodule surface, at least one measurement every 5 mm was performed (mean of the three lower measurements).

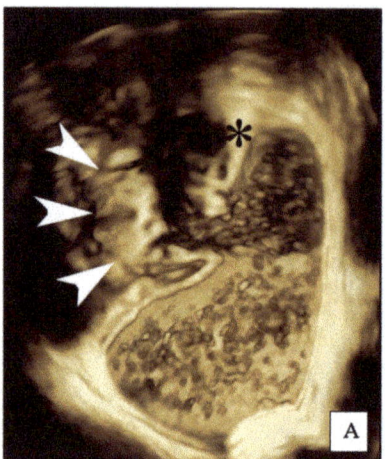 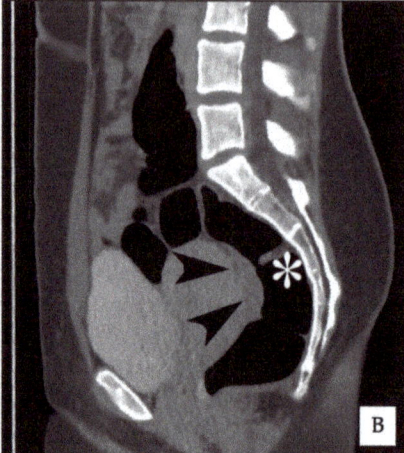

Figure 1. Same rectal endometriotic nodule (arrowheads) is shown in three-dimensional rectal water contrast transvaginal ultrasonography (3D-RWC-TVS) (**A**) and computed tomographic colonography (CTC) (**B**, sagittal plane). The asterisk indicates the same rectal Houston's valve. The nodule has largest diameter of 2.6 cm.

2.2. Computed Colonography

Patients underwent a low residue diet and a liquid diet on the three days before and in the 24 h before CTC, respectively. On the afternoon and the evening of the day before the exam, the patients had an intestinal preparation, which consisted in sodium picosulfate (10.0 mg), light magnesium oxide (3.5 g) and anhydrous citric acid (10.97 g) (CitraFleet, CasenRecordati SL, Zaragoza, Spain). Patients were asked to drink a dose of diatrizoatemeglumine and diatrizoate sodium solution (Gastrografin; Schering, Berlin, Germany) diluted 1:1 with tap water at 6 p.m. on the day before the exam.

A radiologist (E.B.) with extensive experience in the diagnosis of intestinal endometriosis (>500 exams every year) performed all the exams.

The scans were performed by using a 64-section multidetector CT scanner (LightSpeed, GE Healthcare, Milwaukee, WI, USA) according to a standardized protocol [27]. A 12F Foley catheter was introduced into the distal rectum before the scan on the CT bed, and 2.5–3 L of room air were introduced in the colon, calculating the same number of manual pomp inflations in all the distensions. The patients were scanned in the supine and prone positions. No intravenous injection of iodinated contrast medium was employed. The abdomen was scanned as in conventional CTC performed for rectal cancer screening.

The DLP (dose length product) of CTC depended on the length of the abdominal surface of the women that is related to her height. The estimated radiation dose was in the range of 6 mSv. The adaptive statistical iterative reconstruction (ASIR; GE Healthcare) was used to decrease the x-ray dose without a significant loss of image quality.

A weight-based automated tube-current modulation technique was employed with a tube current range of 130–150 mA for patients weighing less than 70 kg in order to decrease the effective radiation dose (abdominal volume acquisition wCTDi = 6–7 mSv). Collimation was 1.25 mm with a helical pitch of 1.375; the reconstruction interval (overlap) was 1 mm. The raw data were transferred to a workstation having a dedicated CTC software package (General Electric ADW 4.2.4, General Electric Medical System, Milwaukee, WT, USA).

Post-processing image editing was performed, being the scans evaluated by various reconstructions: the 3D endo-luminal FT and virtual dissection reconstructions allowed for the visualization of the lumen of the rectum, sigmoid, and the other parts of the colon. 3D images were always used in case of problem solving; the diagnosis was performed on the basis of axial images and multiplanar reconstructions (MPRs).

Rectosigmoid endometriotic nodules appear on CTC as strictures usually involving a variable part of the circumference of the bowel wall (Figure 1); the site of these findings is constant on both the supine and prone scans and stenosis may be highlighted by the 3D endo-luminal FT reconstructions (Figure 2). The MPRs sometimes allow for the detection of a transmural involvement of the endometriotic nodule [27].

For estimating the stenosis, at least one measurement of the diameter of rectosigmoid lumen was performed every 10 mm in the 50 mm above and below the nodule (mean of all measurements) in healthy bowel; on the nodule surface, at least one measurement every 5 mm was performed (mean of the three lower measurements).

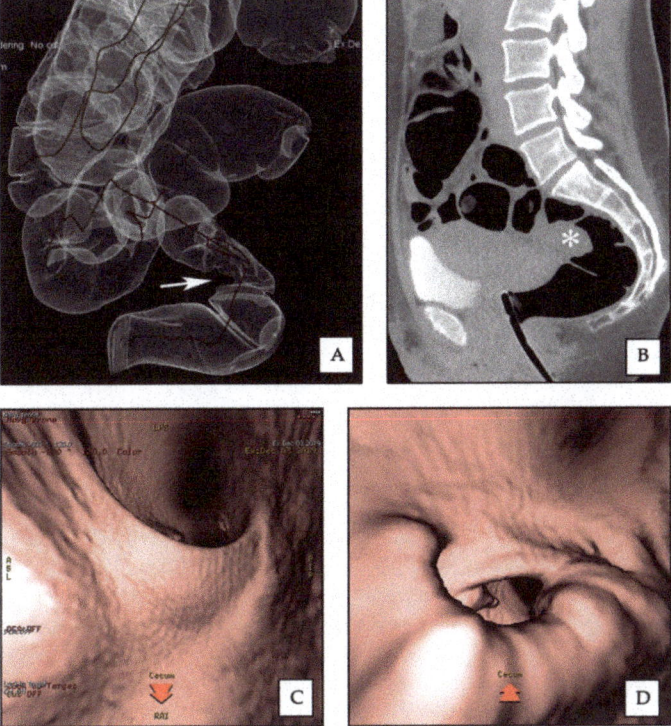

Figure 2. *Cont.*

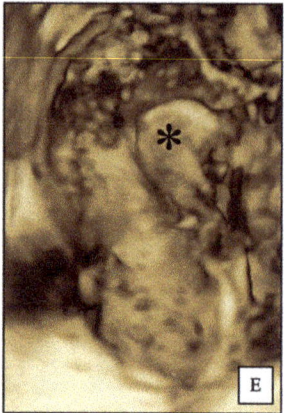

Figure 2. Rectal endometriotic nodule. (**A**) CTC: 3D reconstruction of dilated colon, showing rectal stenosis (arrow) by an endometriotic nodule. (**B**) CTC: sagittal 2D image, the rectal nodule (asterisk) causes stenosis of the intestinal lumen. (**C**) CTC: pseudoendoscopic view and 3D endoluminal fly-through reconstruction, showing normal rectal lumen. (**D**) CTC: pseudoendoscopic view and 3D endoluminal fly-through reconstruction, showing rectal stenosis by the endometriotic nodule. (**E**) 3D-RWC-TVS showing the rectal nodule (asterisk). The nodule has a largest diameter of 2.8 cm; the distance between the lower margin of the nodule and the anal verge is 10 cm.

2.3. Tolerability of Radiological Exams

After each exam, the intensity of the pain perceived was rated by each patient by using a 100-mm visual analogue scale (VAS) scale. Furthermore, patients were asked to qualitatively rate the discomfort perceived during the exam by a 5-point Likert scale (very tolerable, tolerable, neutral, painful, very painful).

2.4. Surgical Procedures

The surgeons were aware of the findings of the 3D-RWC-TVS and CTC. A team of gynecological and colorectal surgeons performed all the procedures by laparoscopy. The rectosigmoid nodules were excised by shaving (excision of the nodule with cold scissor or monopolar hook without entering the intestinal lumen), discoid excision (removal of the nodule with opening of the intestinal wall and suture of the bowel) or by segmental bowel resection. The retrieval of surgical specimens was done through laparoscopic accesses by using an endo-bag (the laparoscopic accesses may have been enlarged in case of large specimen). The morcellation of surgical specimens was always avoided. During laparoscopy, the distance between the main rectosigmoid endometriotic nodule and the anal verge was estimated by introducing a 20-F soft rectal catheter within the rectum up to the level of the intestinal lesion. In case of laparoscopic shaving, a rectal probe was employed for exposing better the endometriotic lesion. In patients who underwent segmental bowel resection, the stenosis of bowel lumen caused by endometriosis was evaluated.

2.5. Statistical Analysis

Accuracy, sensitivity, specificity, positive predictive value (PPV) and negative predictive value (NPV) were evaluated for 3D-RWC-TVS and CTC. The diagnostic value of each technique was also assessed by calculating the positive likelihood ratio and negative likelihood ratio. Efficacy parameters were calculated with 95% confidence intervals (CIs). The accuracy of 3D-RWC-TVS and CTC in the diagnosis of intestinal endometriosis was compared by using the McNemar's test with the Yates continuity correction. The precision of the measurements of nodule size and distance from the anal verge by imaging techniques was calculated by subtracting the size of the nodule, as measured by the imaging techniques, from the size of the nodule, as measured at histology. The limits of agreement were calculated as mean difference ± 2 standard deviations of the difference. Correlations between nominal categories were estimated by phi coefficient. The normality of distribution of continuous variables was evaluated by the Kolmogorov–Smirnov normality test. The pain intensity experienced by the patients during both exams was evaluated by the nonparametric Mann–Whitney test. The data were analyzed using the SPSS software version 24.0 (SPSS Science, Chicago, IL, USA). p values < 0.05 was considered statistically significant.

3. Results

3.1. Characteristics of the Study Population

Table 1 shows the demographic characteristics and Supplementary Table S1 presents the main symptoms complained by the study population. Out of the 68 women included in the study, 37 (48.9; 95% C.I. 38.2–59.7%) had rectosigmoid nodules and underwent bowel surgery. The main nodules were located on the sigmoid in 16 (43.2%) patients, on the rectosigmoid junction in four (10.8%) patients, on the upper rectum in 10 (27.0%) patients and on the lower rectum in seven patients (18.9%). Twelve patients (32.4%) underwent shaving of the colorectal nodules; nine (24.3%) underwent discoid excision; 16 patients (43.2%) underwent segmental colorectal resection; in this last group of patients, the mean (± SD) length of the resected bowel specimen was 11.5 ± 1.9 cm. Concerning the depth of infiltration of endometriosis in the intestinal wall, at histology, the disease infiltrated only the muscularis mucosae in 33 patients (75.0%), the submucosa in eight patients (18.2%) and the mucosa in three patients (6.8%). Seven patients (15.9%) had multifocal disease.

Table 1. Demographic characteristics of the study population (n = 68).

Age (years; mean ± SD)	35.4 ± 6.0
Body mass index (kg/m^2; mean ± SD)	24.7 ± 3.2
Race (n, %)	
• Caucasian	64 (94.1%)
• African	3 (4.4%)
• Asiatic	1 (1.5%)
Previous live birth (n, %)	19 (27.9%)
Previous surgery for endometriosis (n, %)	30 (44.1%)
Concomitant endometriomas (n, %)	32 (47.1%)
Use of hormonal therapies at the time of study inclusion and surgical approach (n, %)	50 (73.5%)
- oral estroprogestin pill	13
- contraceptive vaginal ring	2
- desogestrel	5
- norethindrone acetate	15
- dienogest	9
- etonogestrel-releasing implant	3
- levonorgestrel-releasing intrauterine device	2
- gonadotropin-releasing hormone analogue	1

3.2. Diagnostic Performance of 3D-RTW-TVS and CTC

3D-RTW-TVS and CTC detected 26 (70.3%) and 35 (94.6%) rectosigmoid endometriotic nodules out of 37 confirmed during surgery (Figure 2 and Table 2). There was no significant difference in the accuracy of 3D-RWC-TVS and CTC in diagnosing the presence of rectosigmoid endometriotic nodules (p = 0.118). However, a subgroup analysis demonstrated that CTC was more precise than 3D-RWC-TVS in diagnosing endometriosis located in the sigmoid (p = 0.016). In fact, 3D-RWC-TVS did not identify the presence of eight sigmoid nodules, whereas CTC did not identify only one sigmoid endometriotic nodule. The presence of an endometrioma with diameter >4 cm was positively statistically correlated to the lack of identification of sigmoid endometriotic nodules (phi coefficient 0.516; $p = 0.039$) during 3D-RWC-TVS, but not during CTC (phi coefficient 0.333; $p = 0.182$).

Table 2. Diagnostic performance of 3D-RWC-TVS and CTC in the diagnosis of rectosigmoid endometriosis.

	3D-RWC-TVS	CTC
Sensitivity [a]	70.27% (53.02% to 84.13%)	94.59% (81.81% to 99.34%)
Specificity [a]	96.55% (82.24% to 99.91%)	93.10% (77.23% to 99.15%)
Positive likelihood ratio [b]	20.38 (2.94 to 141.42)	13.72 (3.59 to 52.36)
Negative likelihood ratio [b]	0.31 (0.19 to 0.51)	0.06 (90.02 to 0.22)
Positive predictive value [a]	96.30% (78.93% to 99.45%)	94.59% (82.09% to 98.53%)
Negative predictive value [a]	71.79% (60.69% to 80.76%)	93.10% (77.75% to 98.12%)
Accuracy [a]	81.82% (70.39% to 90.24%)	93.94% (85.20% to 98.32%)

[a] Values presented as percentage and 95% confidence interval; [b] Values presented as ratio and 95% confidence interval; 3D-RWC-TVS: Three-dimensional rectal water contrast transvaginal ultrasonography; CTC: Computed colonography.

The mean (±SD) largest diameter of the main endometriotic nodule at histology was 22.3 (±8.7) mm. 3D-RWC-TVS and CTC estimated the largest diameter of the main endometriotic nodules ($p = 0.099$) similarly, independent of their location. The mean difference was −3.2 (±7.4) mm (95% CI, −6.0 to −0.3 mm; limits of agreement, −17.3 to 11.1 mm) at 3D-RWC-TVS and −1.0 (±2.7) mm (95% CI, −2.1 to 0.1 mm; limits of agreement, −6.4 to 4.5 mm) at CTC when compared with histology (Table 3).

Table 3. Difference between the size of the largest nodule estimated by imaging techniques and that measured on histopathology.

Location	Length on Histology (mm; Mean ±SD)	3D-RWC-TVS		CTC		p [c]
		Difference (mm; mean, 95% CI) [a]	LA [b]	Difference (mm; Mean, 95% CI) [a]	LA [b]	
All ($n = 37$)	22.3 ± 8.7	−3.2 (−6.0 to −0.3)	−17.3 to 11.1	−1.0 (−2.1 to 0.1)	−6.4 to 4.5	0.099
Anterior lower rectum ($n = 7$)	22.1 ± 12.4	−1.0 (−3.3 to 1.4)	−5.5 to 3.3	−1.0 (−3.7 to 1.7)	−6.0 to 4.0	1.000
Anterior upper rectum ($n = 13$)	26.9 ± 11.3	−1.0 (−3.2 to 1.2)	−6.2 to 4.2	−1.3 (−2.7 to 0.2)	−4.4 to 1.7	0.836
Rectosigmoid junction ($n = 4$)	20.3 ± 3.1	1.6 (−3.5 to 6.8)	−2.4 to 5.7	1.0 (−1.5 to 3.5)	−3.1 to 3.6	0.728
Sigmoid ($n = 17$)	22.0 ± 6.4	−7.2 (−15.4 to −3.2)	−16.4 to 9.1	−1.4 (−3.8 to 1.1)	−8.2 to 6.3	0.060

[a] Mean difference calculated by subtracting the size of the nodule measured by the imaging technique from the size of the nodule measured on histology; [b] Limits of agreement (LA) calculated as a mean difference ±2 SDs of the difference. [c] Comparison of the mean difference of 3D-RWC-TVS with that of CTC. 3D-RWC-TVS: Three-dimensional rectal water contrast transvaginal ultrasonography; CTC: Computed colonography

At surgery, the mean (±SD) distance between the more distal rectosigmoid nodule and the anal verge was 142.7 (±45.3) mm. CTC was more accurate than 3D-RWC-TVS in estimating the distance between the lower margin of the intestinal nodule and the anal verge ($p = 0.030$). The mean difference was −16.5 (±30.1) mm (95% CI, −28.7 to −4.2 mm; limits of agreement, −75.7 to 43.4) for 3D-RWC-TVS and 3.3 (±2.0) mm (95% CI, −10.1 to 16.7 mm; limits of agreement, −57.3 to 62.1) for CTC when compared with surgery (Table 4).

Table 4. Difference between the lower margin of the lowest rectosigmoid nodule and the anal verge estimated by imaging techniques and that measured on histopathology.

Location	Distance at Surgery (mm; mean ±SD)	3D-RWC-TVS		CTC		p^c
		Difference (mm; Mean, 95% CI) [a]	LA [b]	Difference (mm; Mean, 95% CI) [a]	LA [b]	
All (n = 37)	142.7 ± 45.3	−16.5 (−28.7 to −4.2)	−75.7 to 43.4	3.3 (−10.1 to 16.7)	−57.3 to 62.1	0.030
Anterior lower rectum (n = 7)	90.7 ± 10.9	3.1 (−14.1 to 20.4)	−28.7 to 32.1	6.6 (−0.1 to 13.4)	−5.9 to 19.2	0.653
Anterior upper rectum (n = 13)	131.3 ± 16.5	−25.6 (−58.2 to 7.1)	−34.8 to 11.0	13.8 (−30.3 to 58.1)	−91.0 to 11.2	0.125
Rectosigmoid junction (n = 4)	138.3 ± 7.6	−6.6 (−32.5 to 19.1)	−27.1 to 13.7	−11.7 (−30.6 to 7.3)	−27.0 to 0.4	0.667
Sigmoid (n = 17)	165.7 ± 47.5	−23.8 (−43.1 to −4.4)	−73.1 to 16.8	−4.5 (−13.4 to 4.5)	−26.3 to 23.0	0.048

[a] Mean difference calculated by subtracting distance between the nodule and anal verge measured by imaging technique from distance between the nodule and anal verge measured at surgery. [b] Limits of agreement (LA) calculated as mean difference ±2 SDs of the difference. [c] Comparison of the mean difference of 3D-RWC-TVS with that of CTC. 3D-RWC-TVS: Three-dimensional rectal water contrast transvaginal ultrasonography; CTC: Computed colonography.

In patients undergoing colorectal segmental resection, at pathological examination, the degree of the stenosis of the bowel lumen was 65.1 (±21.4) %. CTC and 3D-RWC-TVS similarly estimated the degree of the stenosis of the bowel lumen ($p = 0.293$), although 3D-RWC-TVS was less accurate than CTC in determining this parameter in endometriotic nodules located in the sigmoid ($p = 0.005$). The mean difference was 17.3 (±13.8) % for 3D-RWC-TVS and 13.8 (±10.0) % for CTC in comparison to surgery (Figure 3).

CTC only identified all the cases (6/6) of multifocal disease; in one patient, 3D-RWC-TVS did not diagnose the presence of multifocal disease that was diagnosed at surgery (1/6; 16.6%). There was no significant difference in the performance of 3D-RWC-TVS and CTC in diagnosing multifocal disease ($p = 1.000$) (Supplementary Table S2).

The mean (±SD) intensity of pain experienced during CTC was higher than that perceived during RWC-TVS (VAS, 29 ± 57 vs. 15 ± 05 mm; $p < 0.001$). A higher proportion of patients complained of pain during CTC than RWC-TVS (the % of patients experiencing a painful/very painful exam was 7.5% vs. 44.1%; $p < 0.001$).

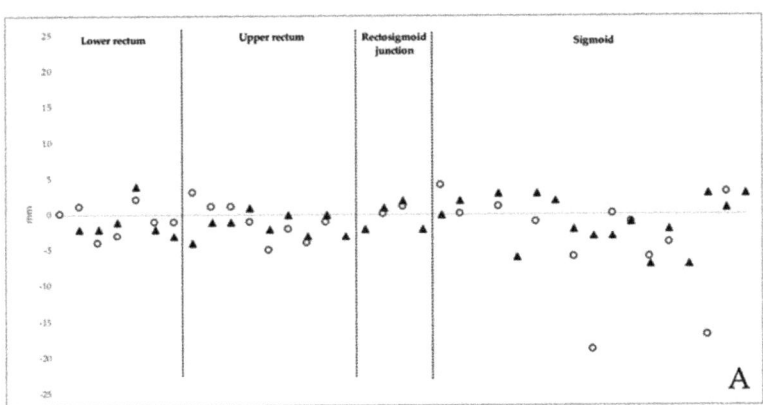

Figure 3. *Cont.*

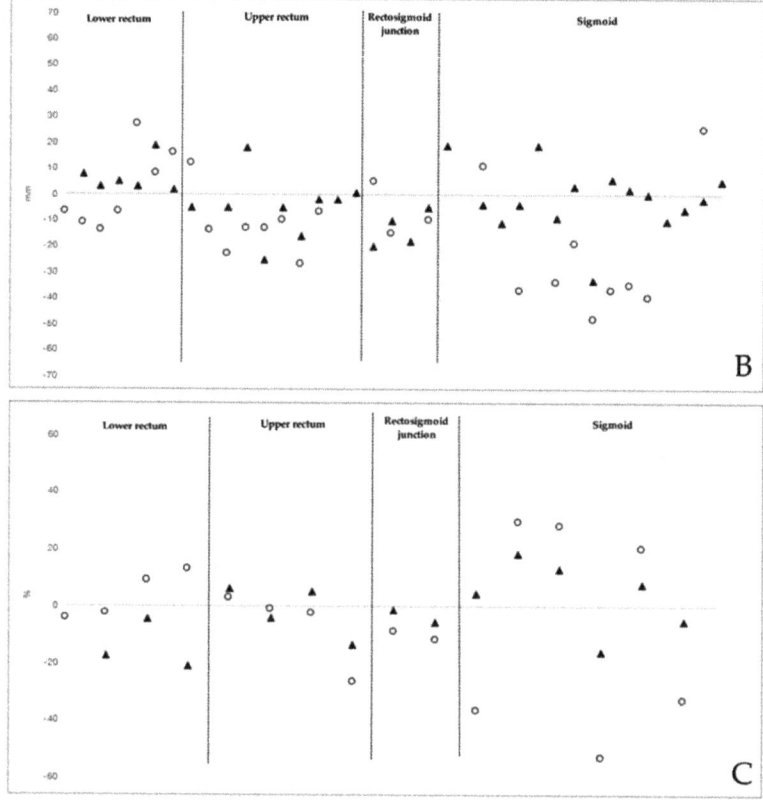

Figure 3. (**A**) Difference (mm) between imaging methods and surgery in estimating the largest diameter of endometriotic rectosigmoid nodules; (**B**) difference (mm) between imaging methods and surgery in estimating the distance from the lowest endometriotic rectosigmoid nodule and the anal verge; (**C**) Difference (%) between imaging methods and surgery in estimating the stenosis of bowel lumen due to the endometriotic nodules (calculated in patients undergoing colorectal segmental resection). White circles: 3D-RWC-TVS; black triangles: CTC.

4. Discussion

This is the first study comparing the performance of 3D-RWC-TVS and CTC in the diagnosis of rectosigmoid endometriosis. Both techniques are based on the distention of the rectosigmoid (with either saline solution or air/CO_2) and allow for the evaluation of the profile of the bowel lumen in a pseudoendoscopic fashion. Moreover, 3D-RWC-TVS and CTC enable the acquisition of ultrasonographic volumetric data with unrestricted access to an infinite number of viewing planes; thus, further images can be obtained even after the first acquisition.

Our data demonstrate that 3D-RWC-TVS and CTC have similar accuracy in the diagnosis of rectosigmoid endometriosis (81.82% vs. 93.94%). However, CTC is more accurate than 3D-RWC-TVS in assessing the presence of sigmoid nodules. In fact, most of the nodules (8/11; 72.7%) not detected by 3D-RWC-TVS were located in the sigmoid; nevertheless, 62.5% of patients (6/10) had ovarian endometriotic cysts with a diameter >4 cm that may have hampered the detection of these upper intestinal nodules. Overall, thirteen false negatives procedures occurred in our study; however, in twelve cases (92.3%), the detection of endometriotic nodules was done by at least one of the two imaging techniques. These data may justify the combined use of both CTC and 3D-RWC-TVS for the workup of patients with suspicion of rectosigmoid endometriosis.

CTC was more precise than 3D-RWC-TVS in estimating the distance between the lower margin of the intestinal nodule and the anal verge: in particular, both techniques equally estimated this parameter in patients with lower, upper rectum, and rectosigmoid junction endometriotic nodules, but not in those with sigmoid nodules. Furthermore, these diagnostic exams were equally precise in estimating the largest diameter of the main rectosigmoid nodule and detecting the presence of multifocal disease.

According to IDEA consensus opinion [6], TVS should be considered the first-line imaging technique for investigating women with suspicion of rectosigmoid endometriosis, in particular, whenever performed by expert ultrasonographers in referral centers specializing in diagnosis of endometriosis. Recently, it has been reported that the need for segmental resection in patients with bowel-infiltrating nodules depends on the degree of muscular layer infiltration and corresponding thickness (muscularis rule) in addition to nodule length and can be accurately identified by preoperative ultrasonographic investigation [5]. Nevertheless, until now, nodule features and threshold values for the choice and timing of either conservative or radical surgical approach for rectosigmoid endometriosis have not been well defined [21]. In current practice, the choice of optimal surgical technique should not depend on only rectosigmoid nodule features, but also on patients' symptoms, age, desire of conception and intention to undergo postoperative hormonal treatment for reducing the risk of disease recurrence. However, the preoperative estimation of the stenosis of rectosigmoid lumen may be helpful in the decision to plan surgery, particularly in infertile patients that may be at risk of bowel occlusion during ovarian stimulation and pregnancy [1]. In our study, CTC and 3D-RWC-TVS similarly estimated the degree of the stenosis of the bowel lumen in patients with rectosigmoid nodules undergoing segmental resection. However, 3D-RWC-TVS was again less accurate than CTC in assessing this parameter in endometriotic nodules located above the rectosigmoid junction.

CTC can characterize endometriotic rectosigmoid nodules and precisely assess the distance between their localization and the anal verge. Colonic distension with air provides a better estimation of digestive tract narrowness than that of any other imaging techniques and allows for an accurate investigation of the whole colon and, in particular, of the intestinal nodules located above the sigmoid colon (such as those on the transverse colon and the cecum) [27]. These nodules cannot be diagnosed by TVS because they are beyond the field of view of the transvaginal probe. In addition, they can also be difficult to detect when performing MR, even in the case of rectal enema (which allows for a less extended retrograde colorectal distension in comparison to CTC) [29]. Considering that more than one-third of cases of bowel lesions are multifocal [30], a complete assessment of the colon is essential to detect all endometriotic lesions for planning the surgical management; in fact, multiple endometriotic nodules on the digestive tract may require multiple segmental bowel resections or disc excisions. Furthermore, CTC is a quick outpatient exam characterized by high spatial resolution, and it allows for scanning the entire abdominal volume within seconds; this may rule out some macroscopic visceral findings (such as cysts, or calcifications) that may be relevant in the differential diagnosis of abdominal pain in patients of reproductive age. Nevertheless, CTC should not be considered as an alternative to TVS or MR, because these imaging techniques can offer a better assessment of deep pelvic endometriosis, ovarian endometriotic cysts, and uterine adenomyosis [31].

Previous studies investigated the performance of CTC in the diagnosis of bowel endometriosis [25,27,32–35]. In a prospective study including 92 women undergoing surgery for deep infiltrating endometriosis, Baggio et al. compared the diagnostic value of TVS, serum Ca125 and CTC [33]. Forty-nine subjects had rectosigmoid endometriosis. CTC had the highest accuracy in detecting bowel involvement with a sensitivity of 68% and a specificity of 67%. However, both TVS and CTC had lower performance than that previously reported by other authors, possibly because of the limited experience of the gynecologists and radiologists in the diagnosis of deep endometriosis. Zannoni et al. compared the performance of TVS and CTC in the diagnosis of rectosigmoid endometriosis in a prospective study including 47 patients with suspicion of rectosigmoid endometriosis [34]. The study showed that TVS has higher accuracy in the diagnosis of intestinal deep infiltrating endometriosis in the rectovaginal septum, rectum and sigma. In contrast, the two techniques had similar accuracy for the diagnosis of overall intestinal deep infiltrating endometriosis. Recently, a systematic review with meta-analysis investigated the performance of CTC by meta-regression, showing a global sensitivity of 93% (95% CI 84–100%) and a specificity of 91% (95% CI 81–100%) [36]. In a prospective study by our academic group, CTC was compared to RWC-TVS in 70 patients with suspicion of rectosigmoid endometriosis, obtaining a similar accuracy in diagnosing endometriotic nodules (sensitivity 90.0% and 94.3%; specificity 92.5% and 92,5%, respectively) [27]. The diagnostic performance of 3D-RWC-TVS reported in the current study is lower than that observed with RWC-TVS. In our experience, obtaining good quality 3D acquisition was more difficult in the sigmoid than in the rectum. Similar to the current data, CTC was previously found to be more precise than RWC-TVS in estimating the distance between the lower margin of the rectosigmoid nodule and the anal verge, but it was less tolerated than RWC-TVS [27].

In our prospective study, CTC was performed without the use of iodinated contrast medium in order to reduce the invasiveness of the exam. For this reason, an accurate estimation of the depth of infiltration of endometriosis in the intestinal wall was not feasible; otherwise, 3D-RWC-TVS reliably estimates this parameter [12].

Ultrasonographic study with 3D modalities has increasingly been employed for the evaluation of many gynecological diseases, being in recent years also investigated for the diagnosis of deep endometriosis [17–19,37]. Two previous studies prospectively compared the performance of 3D-RWC-TVS and MR with colorectal enema in the diagnosis of rectosigmoid endometriosis, finding similar accuracy parameters, nevertheless stating the advantage of an accurate visualization and characterization of the nodules by performing the 3D evaluation [38,39]. In particular, 3D-RWC-TVS is characterized by a wide spatial orientation by providing the observer with a range of different displays of the images in the three orthogonal planes. Moreover, all the acquisitions can be selected and rotated or scrolled through in fascinating virtual navigation and they can be easily assessed off-line. In our study, this advantage let us avoid a 3D real-time evaluation, which would have been subjected to the risk of bias due to 2D-RWC-TVS scan performed at the same consultation; thus, after being stored, the images acquired were interpreted by another expert ultrasonographer blinded to the results of conventional RWC-TVS and CTC imaging. Otherwise, a learning curve has to be considered because the sonographer acquired optimal expertise in 3D acquisitions and interpretation. Notably, the comparison of accuracy of 3D-RWC-TVS versus conventional 2D-RWC-TVS in the detection or characterization of rectosigmoid endometriotic nodules would be of interest. Until now, only a study published in the abstract form performed a preliminary comparison between the two ultrasonographic techniques. This study included 36 women of reproductive age with pain symptoms and intestinal complaints suggestive of rectosigmoid endometriosis. 3D-RWC-TVS and 2D-RWC-TVS had similar performance in the diagnosis of rectosigmoid endometriosis ($p = 0.50$). In particular, for the 3D-RWC-TVS, the sensitivity, specificity, positive and negative predictive values were 86.4%, 85.7%, 90.5% and 80.0%. The two techniques similarly estimated the volume of the largest intestinal nodule and the distance between the lower endometriotic bowel nodule and the anus [40].

In a similar way to the conventional 2D scan, 3D-RWC-TVS is better tolerated and less expensive than CTC. Our data show that patients experienced more discomfort during CTC than during 3D-RWC-TVS. This may be in primis due to the air distension of the colon employed during the radiologic exam, but also to the intestinal cleansing required prior to the exam, less tolerable than that employed for 3D-RWC-TVS. Another not negligible disadvantage related to the use of CTC is the exposure to X-rays; this limit is relevant since women with symptomatic endometriosis are in their fertile age and do not have an oncological pathology that would justify the radiation dose. Nevertheless, in current CTC protocols, the radiation dose has been decreased, and the average radiation administered to the patient is around 6–7 mSv that is lower than that usually used for a barium enema.

This study has some limitations. Indeed, the extensive experience of the radiologist and the gynecologist performing CTC and 3D-RWC-TVS, respectively, may have influenced the accuracy of these techniques in diagnosing rectosigmoid endometriosis. Moreover, we did not perform a power calculation for determining the sample size. As this study was based on a population of symptomatic patients with a high prevalence of intestinal symptoms, a high prevalence of rectosigmoid endometriosis was observed in this sample; subsequently, this issue may potentially have influenced the diagnostic performance of CTC and 3D-RWC-TVS. Nevertheless, the use of these diagnostic exams is justified only in symptomatic patients at high risk of having rectosigmoid endometriosis. The positive, but not statistically significant, trend in favor of CTC with regard to diagnostic parameters may be partly due to limited sample size of our study.

5. Conclusions

In conclusion, 3D-RWC-TVS and CTC can be used to screen the presence of rectosigmoid endometriosis, as they have comparable diagnostic accuracy. However, we deem that symptomatic patients in case of negative findings at 3D-RWC-TVS and patients undergoing surgery should also be investigated using other techniques, aiming to study the presence of sigmoid or upper intestinal nodules. Nevertheless, CTC should not be considered as an alternative to TVS or MR, because these imaging techniques provide a better assessment of deep pelvic endometriosis, ovarian endometriotic cysts, and uterine adenomyosis. In this perspective, CTC may be combined with 3D-RWC-TVS because of the high diagnostic performance in detecting rectosigmoid endometriosis and the ability to diagnose endometriotic nodules located above the sigmoid.

Supplementary Materials: The following are available online at http://www.mdpi.com/2075-4418/10/4/252/s1, Table S1: Presence and intensity of pain and intestinal symptoms in the study population (n = 68), Table S2: Diagnostic performance of 3D-RWC-TVS and CTC in the diagnosis of multifocal rectosigmoid endometriosis

Author Contributions: Conceptualization, F.B. and S.F.; methodology, F.B., F.G. and C.S.(Carolina Scala); software, C.S. (Carolina Scala) and E.B.; validation, F.B., A.S.L.; formal analysis, V.G.V., C.S.(Cesare Stabilini); investigation, E.B., V.G.V., F.B. and S.F.; writing—original draft preparation, F.B.; writing—review and editing, S.F. All authors have read and agreed to the published version of the manuscript.

Funding: This research received no external funding.

Conflicts of Interest: The authors declare no conflict of interest.

References

1. Remorgida, V.; Ferrero, S.; Fulcheri, E.; Ragni, N.; Martin, D.C. Bowel endometriosis: Presentation, diagnosis, and treatment. *Obstet. Gynecol. Surv.* **2007**, *62*, 461–470. [CrossRef]
2. Abrao, M.S.; Petraglia, F.; Falcone, T.; Keckstein, J.; Osuga, Y.; Chapron, C. Deep endometriosis infiltrating the recto-sigmoid: Critical factors to consider before management. *Hum. Reprod. Update* **2015**, *21*, 329–339. [CrossRef]
3. Ferrero, S.; Camerini, G.; Ragni, N.; Venturini, P.L.; Biscaldi, E.; Seracchioli, R.; Remorgida, V. Letrozole and norethisterone acetate in colorectal endometriosis. *Eur. J. Obs. Gynecol. Reprod. Biol.* **2010**, *150*, 199–202. [CrossRef]
4. Ferrero, S.; Camerini, G.; Leone Roberti Maggiore, U.; Venturini, P.L.; Biscaldi, E.; Remorgida, V. Bowel endometriosis: Recent insights and unsolved problems. *World. J. Gastrointest. Surg.* **2011**, *3*, 31–38. [CrossRef]
5. Malzoni, M.; Casarella, L.; Coppola, M.; Falcone, F.; Iuzzolino, D.; Rasile, M.; Di Giovanni, A. Preoperative Ultrasound Indications Determine Excision Technique for Bowel Surgery for Deep Infiltrating Endometriosis: A Single, High-Volume Center. *J. Minim. Invasive. Gynecol.* **2020**. [CrossRef]
6. Guerriero, S.; Condous, G.; van den Bosch, T.; Valentin, L.; Leone, F.P.; Van Schoubroeck, D.; Exacoustos, C.; Installe, A.J.; Martins, W.P.; Abrao, M.S.; et al. Systematic approach to sonographic evaluation of the pelvis in women with suspected endometriosis, including terms, definitions and measurements: A consensus opinion from the International Deep Endometriosis Analysis (IDEA) group. *Ultrasound. Obs. Gynecol.* **2016**, *48*, 318–332. [CrossRef]
7. Takeuchi, H.; Kuwatsuru, R.; Kitade, M.; Sakurai, A.; Kikuchi, I.; Shimanuki, H.; Kinoshita, K. A novel technique using magnetic resonance imaging jelly for evaluation of rectovaginal endometriosis. *Fertil. Steril.* **2005**, *83*, 442–447. [CrossRef]

8. Kikuchi, I.; Takeuchi, H.; Kuwatsuru, R.; Kitade, M.; Kumakiri, J.; Kuroda, K.; Takeda, S. Diagnosis of complete cul-de-sac obliteration (CCDSO) by the MRI jelly method. *J. Magn. Reson. Imaging.* **2009**, *29*, 365–370. [CrossRef]
9. Loubeyre, P.; Petignat, P.; Jacob, S.; Egger, J.F.; Dubuisson, J.B.; Wenger, J.M. Anatomic distribution of posterior deeply infiltrating endometriosis on MRI after vaginal and rectal gel opacification. *Ajr. Am. J. Roentgenol.* **2009**, *192*, 1625–1631. [CrossRef]
10. Chassang, M.; Novellas, S.; Bloch-Marcotte, C.; Delotte, J.; Toullalan, O.; Bongain, A.; Chevallier, P. Utility of vaginal and rectal contrast medium in MRI for the detection of deep pelvic endometriosis. *Eur. Radiol.* **2010**, *20*, 1003–1010. [CrossRef]
11. Biscaldi, E.; Ferrero, S.; Leone Roberti Maggiore, U.; Remorgida, V.; Venturini, P.L.; Rollandi, G.A. Multidetector computerized tomography enema versus magnetic resonance enema in the diagnosis of rectosigmoid endometriosis. *Eur. J. Radiol.* **2014**, *83*, 261–267. [CrossRef]
12. Ferrero, S.; Leone Roberti Maggiore, U.; Barra, F.; Scala, C. Modified ultrasonographic techniques. In *How to Perform Ultrasonography in Endometriosis*; Guerriero, S., Condous, G., Alcazar, J.L., Eds.; Springer: Berlin, Germany, 2018; pp. 133–145.
13. Ferrero, S.; Scala, C.; Stabilini, C.; Vellone, V.G.; Barra, F.; Leone Roberti Maggiore, U. Transvaginal sonography with vs. without bowel preparation in diagnosis of rectosigmoid endometriosis: Prospective study. *Ultrasound. Obs. Gynecol.* **2019**, *53*, 402–409. [CrossRef]
14. Ferrero, S.; Biscaldi, E.; Morotti, M.; Venturini, P.L.; Remorgida, V.; Rollandi, G.A.; Valenzano Menada, M. Multidetector computerized tomography enteroclysis vs. rectal water contrast transvaginal ultrasonography in determining the presence and extent of bowel endometriosis. *Ultrasound. Obstet. Gynecol.* **2011**, *37*, 603–613. [CrossRef]
15. Leone Roberti Maggiore, U.; Biscaldi, E.; Vellone, V.G.; Venturini, P.L.; Ferrero, S. Magnetic resonance enema vs. rectal water-contrast transvaginal sonography in diagnosis of rectosigmoid endometriosis. *Ultrasound. Obs. Gynecol.* **2017**, *49*, 524–532. [CrossRef]
16. Armstrong, L.; Fleischer, A.; Andreotti, R. Three-dimensional volumetric sonography in gynecology: An overview of clinical applications. *Radiol. Clin. N. Am.* **2013**, *51*, 1035–1047. [CrossRef]
17. Guerriero, S.; Alcazar, J.L.; Pascual, M.A.; Ajossa, S.; Perniciano, M.; Piras, A.; Mais, V.; Piras, B.; Schirru, F.; Benedetto, M.G.; et al. Deep Infiltrating Endometriosis: Comparison Between 2-Dimensional Ultrasonography (US), 3-Dimensional US, and Magnetic Resonance Imaging. *J. Ultrasound. Med.* **2018**, *37*, 1511–1521. [CrossRef]
18. Guerriero, S.; Saba, L.; Ajossa, S.; Peddes, C.; Angiolucci, M.; Perniciano, M.; Melis, G.B.; Alcazar, J.L. Three-dimensional ultrasonography in the diagnosis of deep endometriosis. *Hum. Reprod.* **2014**, *29*, 1189–1198. [CrossRef]
19. Grasso, R.F.; Di Giacomo, V.; Sedati, P.; Sizzi, O.; Florio, G.; Faiella, E.; Rossetti, A.; Del Vescovo, R.; Zobel, B.B. Diagnosis of deep infiltrating endometriosis: Accuracy of magnetic resonance imaging and transvaginal 3D ultrasonography. *Abdom. Imaging* **2010**, *35*, 716–725. [CrossRef]
20. Mabrouk, M.; Raimondo, D.; Altieri, M.; Arena, A.; Del Forno, S.; Moro, E.; Mattioli, G.; Iodice, R.; Seracchioli, R. Surgical, Clinical, and Functional Outcomes in Patients with Rectosigmoid Endometriosis in the Gray Zone: 13-Year Long-Term Follow-up. *J. Minim. Invasive. Gynecol.* **2019**, *26*, 1110–1116. [CrossRef]
21. Donnez, O.; Roman, H. Choosing the right surgical technique for deep endometriosis: Shaving, disc excision, or bowel resection? *Fertil. Steril.* **2017**, *108*, 931–942. [CrossRef]
22. Tzambouras, N.; Katsanos, K.H.; Tsili, A.; Papadimitriou, K.; Efremidis, S.; Tsianos, E.V. CT colonoscopy for obstructive sigmoid endometriosis: A new technique for an old problem. *Eur. J. Intern. Med.* **2002**, *13*, 274–275.
23. Van der Wat, J.; Kaplan, M.D. Modified virtual colonoscopy: A noninvasive technique for the diagnosis of rectovaginal septum and deep infiltrating pelvic endometriosis. *J. Minim. Invasive Gynecol.* **2007**, *14*, 638–643. [CrossRef]
24. Koutoukos, I.; Langebrekke, A.; Young, V.; Qvigstad, E. Imaging of endometriosis with computerized tomography colonography. *Fertil. Steril.* **2011**, *95*, 259–260. [CrossRef]
25. Jeong, S.Y.; Chung, D.J.; Myung Yeo, D.; Lim, Y.T.; Hahn, S.T.; Lee, J.M. The usefulness of computed tomographic colonography for evaluation of deep infiltrating endometriosis: Comparison with magnetic resonance imaging. *J. Comput. Assist. Tomogr.* **2013**, *37*, 809–814. [CrossRef]

26. Van der Wat, J.; Kaplan, M.D.; Roman, H.; Da Costa, C. The use of modified virtual colonoscopy to structure a descriptive imaging classification with implied severity for rectogenital and disseminated endometriosis. *J. Minim. Invasive. Gynecol.* **2013**, *20*, 543–546. [CrossRef]
27. Ferrero, S.; Biscaldi, E.; Vellone, V.G.; Venturini, P.L.; Leone Roberti Maggiore, U. Computed tomographic colonography vs. rectal water—Contrast transvaginal sonography in diagnosis of rectosigmoid endometriosis: A pilot study. *Ultrasound. Obs. Gynecol.* **2017**, *49*, 515–523. [CrossRef]
28. Valenzano Menada, M.; Remorgida, V.; Abbamonte, L.H.; Nicoletti, A.; Ragni, N.; Ferrero, S. Does transvaginal ultrasonography combined with water-contrast in the rectum aid in the diagnosis of rectovaginal endometriosis infiltrating the bowel? *Hum. Reprod.* **2008**, *23*, 1069–1075. [CrossRef]
29. Biscaldi, E.; Barra, F.; Ferrero, S. Magnetic Resonance Enema in Rectosigmoid Endometriosis. *Magn. Reson. Imaging Clin. N. Am.* **2020**, *28*, 89–104. [CrossRef]
30. Chapron, C.; Fauconnier, A.; Vieira, M.; Barakat, H.; Dousset, B.; Pansini, V.; Vacher-Lavenu, M.C.; Dubuisson, J.B. Anatomical distribution of deeply infiltrating endometriosis: Surgical implications and proposition for a classification. *Hum. Reprod.* **2003**, *18*, 157–161. [CrossRef]
31. Exacoustos, C.; Manganaro, L.; Zupi, E. Imaging for the evaluation of endometriosis and adenomyosis. *Best. Pr. Res. Clin. Obs. Gynaecol.* **2014**, *28*, 655–681. [CrossRef]
32. Roman, H.; Carilho, J.; Da Costa, C.; De Vecchi, C.; Suaud, O.; Monroc, M.; Hochain, P.; Vassilieff, M.; Savoye-Collet, C.; Saint-Ghislain, M. Computed tomography-based virtual colonoscopy in the assessment of bowel endometriosis: The surgeon's point of view. *Gynecol. Obs. Fertil.* **2016**, *44*, 3–10. [CrossRef]
33. Baggio, S.; Zecchin, A.; Pomini, P.; Zanconato, G.; Genna, M.; Motton, M.; Montemezzi, S.; Franchi, M. The Role of Computed Tomography Colonography in Detecting Bowel Involvement in Women With Deep Infiltrating Endometriosis: Comparison With Clinical History, Serum Ca125, and Transvaginal Sonography. *J. Comput. Assist. Tomogr.* **2016**, *40*, 886–891. [CrossRef]
34. Zannoni, L.; Del Forno, S.; Coppola, F.; Papadopoulos, D.; Valerio, D.; Golfieri, R.; Caprara, G.; Paradisi, R.; Seracchioli, R. Comparison of transvaginal sonography and computed tomography-colonography with contrast media and urographic phase for diagnosing deep infiltrating endometriosis of the posterior compartment of the pelvis: A pilot study. *Jpn. J. Radiol.* **2017**, *35*, 546–554. [CrossRef]
35. Mehedintu, C.; Brinduse, L.A.; Bratila, E.; Monroc, M.; Lemercier, E.; Suaud, O.; Collet-Savoye, C.; Roman, H. Does Computed Tomography-Based Virtual Colonoscopy Improve the Accuracy of Preoperative Assessment Based on Magnetic Resonance Imaging in Women Managed for Colorectal Endometriosis? *J. Minim. Invasive Gynecol.* **2018**. [CrossRef]
36. Woo, S.; Suh, C.H.; Kim, H. Diagnostic performance of computed tomography for bowel endometriosis: A systematic review and meta-analysis. *Eur. J. Radiol.* **2019**, *119*, 108638. [CrossRef]
37. Pascual, M.A.; Guerriero, S.; Hereter, L.; Barri-Soldevila, P.; Ajossa, S.; Graupera, B.; Rodriguez, I. Diagnosis of endometriosis of the rectovaginal septum using introital three-dimensional ultrasonography. *Fertil. Steril.* **2010**, *94*, 2761–2765. [CrossRef]
38. Sandre, A.; Philip, C.A.; De-Saint-Hilaire, P.; Maissiat, E.; Bailly, F.; Cortet, M.; Dubernard, G. Comparison of three-dimensional rectosonography, rectal endoscopic sonography and magnetic resonance imaging performances in the diagnosis of rectosigmoid endometriosis. *Eur. J. Obs. Gynecol. Reprod. Biol.* **2019**, *240*, 288–292. [CrossRef]
39. Philip, C.A.; Prouvot, C.; Cortet, M.; Bisch, C.; de Saint-Hilaire, P.; Maissiat, E.; Huissoud, C.; Dubernard, G. Diagnostic Performances of Tridimensional Rectosonography and Magnetic Resonance Imaging in Rectosigmoid Endometriosis: A Prospective Cohort Study on 101 Patients. *Ultrasound. Med. Biol.* **2019**. [CrossRef]
40. Barra, F.S.; Vellone, V.G.; Ferrero, S. Bidimensional rectal-water contrast-transvaginal ultrasonography (2D-RWC-TVS) versus 3D-RWC-TVS in the diagnosis of rectosigmoid endometriosis: A pilot prospective comparative study. In Proceedings of the ESHRE Annual Meeting, Vienna, Austria, 26–29 June 2019.

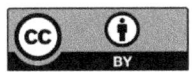

© 2020 by the authors. Licensee MDPI, Basel, Switzerland. This article is an open access article distributed under the terms and conditions of the Creative Commons Attribution (CC BY) license (http://creativecommons.org/licenses/by/4.0/).

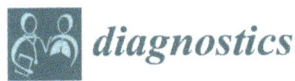

Article

Assessment of Coagulation Parameters in Women Affected by Endometriosis: Validation Study and Systematic Review of the Literature

Jessica Ottolina [1], Ludovica Bartiromo [1], Carolina Dolci [1], Noemi Salmeri [1], Matteo Schimberni [1], Roberta Villanacci [1], Paola Viganò [2,*] and Massimo Candiani [1]

1. Gynecology/Obstetrics Unit, IRCCS San Raffaele Scientific Institute, 20132 Milan, Italy; ottolina.jessica@hsr.it (J.O.); bartiromo.ludovica@hsr.it (L.B.); dolci.carolina@hsr.it (C.D.); salmeri.noemi@hsr.it (N.S.); schimberni.matteo@hsr.it (M.S.); villanacci.roberta@hsr.it (R.V.); candiani.massimo@hsr.it (M.C.)
2. Reproductive Sciences Lab, Division of Genetics and Cell Biology, IRCCS San Raffaele Scientific Institute, 20132 Milan, Italy
* Correspondence: vigano.paola@hsr.it; Tel.: +39-02-26436228; Fax: +39-02-26345266

Received: 21 July 2020; Accepted: 5 August 2020; Published: 7 August 2020

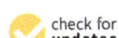

Abstract: The presence of endometriosis determines an inflammatory response locally. The objective of this validation study and systematic review was to assess systemic levels of coagulation and inflammatory parameters in women with or without the disease. We conducted a retrospective analysis of a database prospectively collected from January 2017 to February 2020 including $n = 572$ women who underwent laparoscopic surgery for endometriosis (cases, $n = 324$) or other benign gynecologic diseases (controls, $n = 248$). Inflammatory markers and coagulation parameters were determined. An advanced systematic search of the literature on the same parameters was conducted up to April 2020. A significantly higher neutrophil count was found in endometriosis patients. Patients with endometriomas and stage III–IV disease had a significantly lower absolute lymphocyte count and shortened activated partial thromboplastin time (aPTT) values. In the final regression model, aPTT retained significant predictive value for stage III–IV endometriosis (odds ratio (OR) = 0.002, 95% confidence interval (CI) = 0.00–0.445; $p = 0.024$). Results from the $n = 14$ included studies in the systematic review are characterized by a high variability, but some consistency has been found for alterations in thrombin time, platelet-to-lymphocyte ratio, and neutrophil count associated with endometriosis. Modest systemic changes of some inflammatory and coagulation parameters are associated with endometriosis. Indeed, all the modifications detected are still within the normal reference intervals, explaining the high heterogeneity among studies.

Keywords: endometriosis; coagulation; thrombin time; activated partial thromboplastin time; platelet-to-lymphocyte ratio; neutrophil-to-lymphocyte ratio

1. Introduction

Endometriosis, defined as the presence of endometrial tissue and fibrosis located outside the uterine cavity, is a common chronic disease that affects around 10% of women of reproductive age and is associated with infertility and pelvic pain [1–4]. Traditionally defined as a hormonal disease with an increased local production of estrogens due to aberrant steroidogenesis, it is also characterized by features of a pelvic chronic inflammatory condition. The presence of ectopic tissue in the peritoneal cavity is associated with overproduction of pro-inflammatory and pro-fibrotic cytokines and chemokines (i.e., interleukin (IL)-1β, IL-6, tumor necrosis factor (TNF)-α, and transforming growth factor-β (TGF-β)) detected in endometriotic lesions, endometriotic cyst fluid, and peritoneal fluid [5–8].

Macrophages infiltrating the ectopic lesions express typical markers of alternative activation, favoring the growth of the lesions and promoting their angiogenesis. Some inflammatory parameters, such as the neutrophil-to-lymphocyte ratio (NLR), have also been found elevated in the peripheral blood in patients with some forms of the disease [9,10]. The close association of inflammatory conditions and coagulatory processes has been known for a long time [11]. Platelets are the first immunomodulatory cells at the site of injury and inflammation, providing a functional link between host response and coagulation. Monocytes and neutrophils contribute to coagulation by the expression of tissue factor [7,8], which is upregulated upon inflammation. Other cells of the circulation and vasculature are altered by inflammatory conditions toward a pro-thrombotic state, as well. Moreover, in their activated state, neutrophils are capable of expelling neutrophil extracellular traps, which exert antibacterial functions, but also induce a strong coagulatory response. In line with the presence of a cross-talk between these two systems, platelet count (PLC) has been found to be increased in patients affected by endometriosis [12,13], while activated partial thromboplastin time (aPTT) and thrombin time (TT) were shown to be shortened [12,14]. In 2018, our group specifically demonstrated that endometriosis patients had a significantly shorter aPTT than women not affected by the disease and, in the subgroup analysis, women with ovarian disease had significantly shortened aPTT values in comparison to women without this form. Furthermore, both platelet-to-lymphocyte ratio (PLR) and aPTT were shown to be altered in the less severe forms. Since endometriotic cells express tissue factor (TF), these alterations were suggested to represent the subtle manifestation of the activation of this factor in the lesions and were portrayed in the context of angiogenesis and, thus, the development and progression of the disease [15]. Based on this evidence, coagulation and inflammatory parameters have also been proposed as systemic biomarkers for the presence of endometriosis. However, although their values seem to be significantly different from controls, they still remain in the normal range. In light of these data, other evidence is needed in order to confirm the presence of subtle alterations of coagulation parameters in endometriosis before setting up investigations on the pathogenetic and clinical significance of these findings. We have herein analyzed systemic levels of coagulation and inflammatory parameters in a validation study including women with or without endometriosis undergoing gynecologic pelvic surgery. In addition, to offer a general view of available data, we systematically reviewed and compared our findings with results from the current literature focused on this topic.

2. Materials and Methods

2.1. Retrospective Case–Control Study

This study was based on a retrospective analysis of a surgical database prospectively collected from January 2017 to February 2020 at San Raffaele Scientific Institute in Milan, Italy. All patients had a surgical indication for gynecologic diseases and underwent laparoscopic surgery. All participants met the following inclusion criteria: non-pregnant, reproductive-age women; normal hepatic and renal function tests; and a surgical indication for endometriosis or other benign gynecologic diseases. Women with coagulation disorders, autoimmune diseases, diagnosis of uterine or ovarian malignancy, or concomitant use of antiplatelet or anticoagulant therapy at the time of surgery were excluded. Women whose data on coagulation status were not available were also excluded. Information about age, body mass index (BMI), smoking status, medical history, previous history of gynecological surgery, intraoperative findings, histopathological diagnosis, and routine blood tests were collected. The routine preoperative tests included complete blood count parameters, NLR, PLR, PT (prothrombin time) ratio, aPTT ratio, and international normalized ratio (INR). A peripheral blood sample (2 mL) was obtained from the median cubital vein of each patient and mixed with 3.2% citric acid for anticoagulation purposes. All blood analyses were obtained at a maximum of 1 month before surgery. The NLR was obtained by dividing the absolute neutrophil count by the absolute lymphocyte count, while the PLR was obtained by dividing the absolute platelet count by the absolute lymphocyte count. All blood analyses were done during either the follicular or the luteal phase of the cycle before surgery. The case group included patients with a diagnosis of endometriosis. The stage of endometriosis was established according to the revised American Fertility Society (r-AFS) classification [16]. Endometriotic lesions were classified according to their phenotype as ovarian endometrioma (OMA), deep infiltrating endometriosis (DIE), and superficial peritoneal endometriosis (SPE) [17]. Since these phenotypes are frequently combined, patients were assigned to the group corresponding to the most severe lesion detected, with the severity scale going from the least to the most severe as follows: SPE, OMA, DIE. The control group consisted of women with a surgical diagnosis of tubal pathology and ovarian benign cysts. Both the surgical and the histopathological examinations confirmed no evidence of endometriosis in the control population. According to the abovementioned selection criteria, $n = 572$ women were included: $n = 324$ had a diagnosis of endometriosis, and $n = 248$ had a diagnosis of other gynecologic diseases. All the women signed a written informed consent to record their data for scientific purposes. The Institutional Review Board of our Institution approved the study (Comitato Etico Ospedale San Raffaele; No. 01END, approved 12 April 2012).

2.2. Systematic Review of the Literature

The study was registered and accepted for inclusion in the database PROSPERO (ID CRD42020171524). The systematic review was carried out in accordance with the methods proposed by Preferred Reporting Item for Systematic Reviews and Meta-analysis (PRISMA) guidelines [18]. We performed an advanced, systematic search of online medical databases PubMed and Medline using the following keywords: "endometriosis" in combination with "thrombin", "thrombin time", "thromboplastin", "partial thromboplastin time", "activated partial thromboplastin time", "INR", "international normalized ratio", "coagulation/blood coagulation", "platelets/blood platelets", "lymphocyte", "platelets-to-lymphocyte ratio/platelets-lymphocyte ratio", or "neutrophil-to-lymphocyte ratio/ neutrophil-lymphocyte ratio". To optimize search output, we used specific tools available in each database, such as Medical Subject Headings (MeSH) terms (PubMed/Medline). The EndNote software (available online: https://endnote.com, accessed on 31 May 2020) was used to remove duplicate articles. Only full-length manuscripts written in English up to April 2020 were considered. We checked all citations found by title and abstract to establish the eligibility of the source and obtained the full text of eligible articles. We also performed a manual scan of the references list of the review articles to identify any additional relevant citations. Three review authors (J.O., M.S., and L.B.) independently assessed the risk of bias for each study using the risk-of-bias tool for case–control studies developed by clarity group [19]. We assessed the risk of bias according to the following domains: i) Can we be confident in the assessment of exposure?; ii) Can we be confident that cases had developed the outcome of interest and controls had not?; iii) Were the cases properly selected?; iv) Were the controls properly selected?; v) Were cases and controls matched according to important prognostic variables or was statistical adjustment carried out for those variables?. We graded each potential source of bias as Definitely yes (low risk of bias), Probably yes (Moderate risk of bias), Probably no (Serious risk of bias), or Definitely no (Critical, high risk of bias). We summarized the risk of bias judgments across different studies for each of the domains listed.

2.3. Statistical Analysis

Statistical analysis was performed using IBM SPSS Statistics, Version Chicago 24.0 (IBM Corp. Realesd 2016. Version 24.0. Armonk, NY, USA). Differences in systemic inflammatory response markers between cases and controls were investigated. Coagulation parameters were analyzed including only patients who were not taking any hormonal therapy at the time of surgery. Categorical variables were expressed as absolute value and percentages, and between-groups comparisons were evaluated using the Pearson's chi square test with a Monte Carlo approximation at 95% confidence interval (CI). Continuous and normally distributed variables were presented as mean, range, and standard deviation (SD), and between-groups differences were investigated using the independent Student's t-test. Subgroup analyses according to the stage and type of endometriosis were performed using the one-way analysis of variance (ANOVA) test. Before conducting means comparisons, the assumption of homogeneity of variances was tested and satisfied based on Levene's F tests. In order to evaluate the nature of the differences between the means further, each statistically significant ANOVA test was followed-up with a Bonferroni's post hoc test. A binary logistic regression was conducted in order to evaluate coagulation and inflammatory parameters as independent predictor factors of endometriosis. Adjusted odds ratios with 95% CI were evaluated when a statistically significant correlation was found. p-values < 0.05 were considered statistically significant.

3. Results

3.1. Results of the Retrospective Analysis

Of the $n = 324$ women affected by endometriosis, $n = 85$ were stage I or II (26.2%) disease, whereas the remaining $n = 239$ patients (73.76%) were stages III or IV. According to the type of disease, $n = 214$ patients (66%) were classified as having OMA, $n = 69$ patients (21.3%) as having DIE, and $n = 41$ patients (12.7%) as having SPE. Endometriosis could not be detected in $n = 248$ women. These cases were used as controls. The main diagnosis of this group was as follows: ovarian dermoids ($n = 110$), serous or seromucinous ovarian cysts ($n = 77$), tubal pathology ($n = 43$), and normal pelvis ($n = 18$). The baseline characteristics of patients with and without endometriosis are shown in Table 1.

Table 1. Baseline characteristics of the endometriosis and control groups.

Baseline Characteristics	Endometriosis Group ($n = 324$)	Control Group ($n = 248$)	p-Value
Age (years)	33.53 ± 5.51	31.15 ± 7.9	**0.001**
BMI (kg/m^2)	21.37 ± 3.9	22.29 ± 4.0	**0.028**
Smoking habit	28 (14.7%)	35 (18.3%)	0.09
Indication for surgery			
Symptoms	174 (55.4%)	69 (29%)	
Offspring desire	113 (36%)	56 (23.5%)	**0.001**
Occasional findings	12 (3.8%)	104 (43.7%)	
Symptoms and offspring desire	15 (4.8%)	8 (3.4%)	
Prophylactic surgery		1 (0.4%)	
HT before surgery	128 (39.5%)	64 (25.8%)	0.43
Previous pelvic surgery	82 (25.9%)	85 (34.6%)	**0.027**

Note: values are mean ± SD or absolute value (%). Abbreviations: BMI, body mass index; HT, hormonal therapy. p-values < 0.05 were considered statistically significant (bold values).

In line with previous observations [20], patients with endometriosis had a significantly lower BMI compared with controls; moreover, patients with endometriosis were older than non-endometriosis patients. Results from comparisons of systemic inflammatory parameters between cases and controls are reported in Table 2. A significantly higher neutrophil count was found in patients with endometriosis when compared to controls. No difference in lymphocytes count and NLR was detected between the two groups. When we considered the various manifestations of endometriosis separately, we found that women with ovarian disease had a borderline significant lower absolute lymphocyte count in comparison with controls, SPE group, and DIE group. In addition, women with stage III to IV disease had a slightly lower lymphocyte count than those with stage I to II disease, and the difference reached statistical significance. In order to evaluate the real effect of endometriosis on the coagulation status, we decided to include in the comparisons only cases ($n = 163$) and controls ($n = 96$) who were not taking any hormonal therapy at the time of surgery because of the well-known impact of the treatment on the coagulation parameters [21,22]. Intergroups differences of coagulation parameters and inflammatory response markers in patients without hormonal therapy are shown in Table 3.

Table 2. Systemic inflammatory response parameters according to the different stage and type of endometriosis versus controls.

Diagnosis	L (10^9/L)	N (10^9/L)	NLR
Endometriosis (n = 324)	2.05 ± 0.53	4.30 ± 1.51	2.21 ± 0.95
Controls (n = 248)	2.12 ± 0.55	4.03 ± 1.57	2.05 ± 1.50
	p = 0.13	**p = 0.038**	p = 0.13
OMA (n = 214)	2.01 ± 0.52	4.32 ± 1.51	2.27 ± 0.97
DIE (n = 69)	2.19 ± 0.64	4.36 ± 1.51	2.12 ± 0.95
SPE (n = 41)	2.04 ± 0.56	4.08 ± 1.55	2.04 ± 0.78
Controls (n = 248)	2.12 ± 0.55	4.03 ± 1.57	2.05 ± 1.50
	p = 0.049	p = 0.15	p = 0.27
Stage I–II (n = 85)	2.16 ± 0.56	4.29 ± 1.49	2.06 ± 0.81
Stage III–IV (n = 239)	2.01 ± 0.52	4.30 ± 1.52	2.25 ± 0.99
Controls (n = 248)	2.12 ± 0.55	4.03 ± 1.57	2.05 ± 1.50
	p = 0.032	p = 0.11	p = 0.15

Note: values are mean ± SD or absolute value (%). Abbreviations: OMA, ovarian endometrioma; DIE, deep infiltrating endometriosis; SPE, superficial peritoneal endometriosis; N, neutrophil count; L, lymphocyte count; NLR, neutrophil-to-lymphocyte ratio. p-values < 0.05 were considered statistically significant (bold values).

For inflammatory parameters, in line with the above reported results, patients with OMAs had significantly lower absolute lymphocytes count if compared to both controls and DIE group. No difference in neutrophils count and NLR was detected among the endometriosis phenotypes. Focusing on the coagulation parameters, a significant between-group difference emerged in aPTT values, as women with OMA disease had shortened aPTT values if compared to patients with SPE, DIE, and controls. Moreover, women with stage III–IV disease had slightly, but significantly, shorter aPTT values than those with stage I–II endometriosis or than controls. No difference was found for platelet count or PLR among the various groups. Boxplots of levels of coagulation parameters and systemic inflammatory response markers according to the different stages of endometriosis are presented in Figure 1. A logistic regression was conducted in order to evaluate whether a certain coagulation or inflammatory status could be a predictor of the disease. The binary logistic regression was able to correctly classify 78.5% of cases (R^2 = 0.05, $\chi^2(1)$ = 5.29, p = 0.021). In the final regression model, aPTT retained significant predictive value for stages III–IV endometriosis (b = −6.091, standard error (SE) = 2.695; OR = 0.002, 95% CI = 0.00–0.445; p = 0.024) (Table 4).

Table 3. Coagulation parameters and systemic inflammatory response markers according to the different stage and type of endometriosis versus controls, excluding patients taking hormonal drugs.

Diagnosis	PT Ratio	aPTT Ratio	INR	PLC (10^9/L)	L (10^9/L)	N (10^9/L)	NLR	PLR
OMA (n = 118)	1.05 ± 0.06	1.01 ± 0.07	1.06 ± 0.07	253.5 ± 62.0	1.93 ± 0.49	3.99 ± 1.48	2.18 ± 1.03	69.81 ± 25.6
DIE (n = 28)	1.05 ± 0.06	1.05 ± 0.08	1.05 ± 0.07	268.7 ± 73.0	2.29 ± 0.64	3.96 ± 1.27	1.79 ± 0.60	72.43 ± 22.7
SPE (n = 17)	1.07 ± 0.09	1.04 ± 0.07	1.07 ± 0.12	254.5 ± 53.1	1.97 ± 0.33	3.51 ± 1.26	1.80 ± 0.63	81.43 ± 33.0
Controls (n = 96)	1.05 ± 0.06	1.03 ± 0.06	1.06 ± 0.06	249.4 ± 50.2	2.11 ± 0.49	3.99 ± 1.57	1.99 ± 0.96	72.93 ± 37.6
	p = 0.61	p = 0.049	p = 0.59	p = 0.50	p = **0.003** [b]	p = 0.64	p = 0.117	p = 0.52
Stage I–II (n = 35)	1.06 ± 0.08	1.05 ± 0.08	1.06 ± 0.09	262.3 ± 64.7	2.12 ± 0.59	3.77 ± 1.36	1.83 ± 0.62	76.55 ± 27.4
Stage III–IV (n = 128)	1.02 ± 0.07	1.01 ± 0.07	1.06 ± 0.06	254.6 ± 62.8	1.97 ± 0.49	3.98 ± 1.45	2.14 ± 1.01	70.09 ± 25.6
Controls (n = 96)	1.05 ± 0.06	1.03 ± 0.06	1.06 ± 0.06	249.4 ± 50.2	2.11 ± 0.49	3.99 ± 1.57	1.99 ± 0.96	72.93 ± 37.6
	p = 0.78	p = **0.040** [b]	p = 0.82	p = 0.53	p = 0.07	p = 0.73	p = 0.18	p = 0.51

Note: values are mean ± SD or absolute value (%). Abbreviations: OMA, ovarian endometrioma; DIE, deep infiltrating endometriosis; SPE, superficial peritoneal endometriosis; PT, prothrombin time; aPTT, activated partial thromboplastin time; INR, international normalized ratio; PLC, platelet count; N, neutrophil count; L, lymphocyte count; NLR, neutrophil-to-lymphocyte ratio; PLR, platelet-to-lymphocyte ratio. [b] When p < 0.05, a Bonferroni's post hoc test was performed for within-groups differences. p-values < 0.05 were considered statistically significant (bold values).

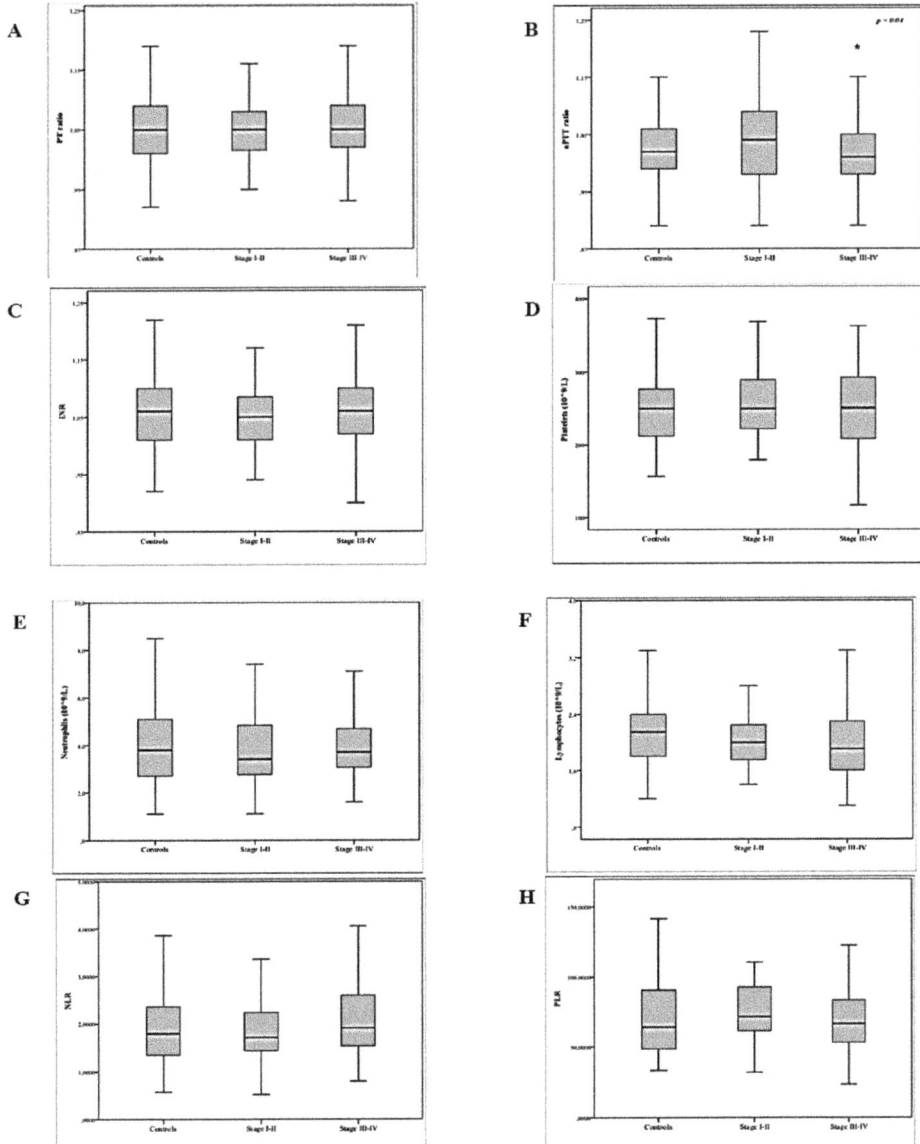

Figure 1. Boxplots of levels of coagulation parameters and systemic inflammatory response parameters according to different stages of endometriosis (n = 259). (**A**) PT, prothrombin time; (**B**) aPTT, activated partial thromboplastin time; (**C**) INR, international normalized ratio; (**D**) PLC, platelet count; (**E**) N, neutrophil count; (**F**) L, lymphocyte count; (**G**) NLR, neutrophil-to-lymphocyte ratio; (**H**) PLR, platelet-to-lymphocyte ratio. * p = 0.04.

Table 4. Logistic regression of coagulation and inflammatory parameters predicting the stage of endometriosis.

Variable	B Coefficient	SE	OR	p-Value
PT ratio	−4.084	12.301		0.74
aPTT ratio	−6.091	2.695	0.002	0.024
INR	3.611	11.279		0.75
PLC (10^9/L)	0.000	0.006		0.95
L (10^9/L)	−0.587	0.728		0.42
N (10^9/L)	0.645	1.355		0.63
NLR	1.342	1.402		0.34
PLR	−0.007	0.018		0.71

Abbreviations: SE, standard error; OR, odds ratio; PT, prothrombin time; aPTT, activated partial thromboplastin time; INR, international normalized ratio; PLC, platelet count; N, neutrophil count; L, lymphocyte count; NLR, neutrophil-to-lymphocyte ratio; PLR, platelet-to-lymphocyte ratio. p-values < 0.05 were considered statistically significant (bold values).

3.2. Results of the Systematic Review

The search revealed $n = 17$ studies eligible for inclusion in this systematic review. Of these, $n = 14$ were finally included [9,12–14,23–32]. A flow diagram of the systematic review is shown in Figure 2 (PRISMA template). The main characteristics of the included studies are summarized in Table 5. The risks of bias of the included studies are summarized in Supplementary Figure S1.

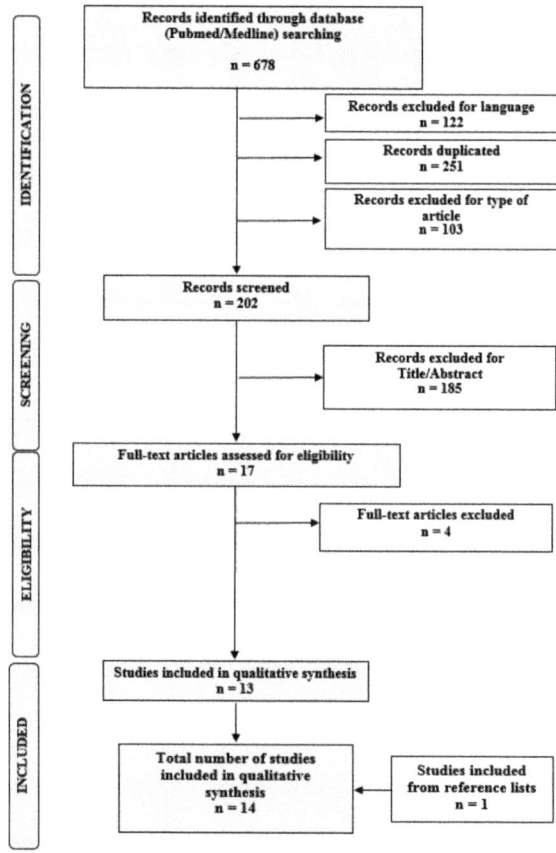

Figure 2. Flow diagram of the search strategy, screening, eligibility, and inclusion criteria.

Table 5. Main characteristics of considered studies.

Author, Years	Country	Study Design	Study Period	Cases/Controls Sample Size (n)	Age (Years)	Parameters Assessed (When)	Confounding Factors
Cho et al., 2008 [23]	South Korea	Retrospective case-control study	01/2004 12/2007	Endometriosis [1] (231)/ Benign ovarian cysts [1] (231) Healthy women [2] (384)	33.3 ± 7.3 * (Overall) 32.6 ± 7.35 * (endometriosis) 34.2 ± 8.9 * (benign ovarian cyst) 33.9 ± 5.7 * (healthy women)	Complete blood cell count, NLR, and CA125 (before surgery or as part of routine health examination [3])	Unclear
Yavuzcan et al., 2013 [25]	Turkey	Retrospective case-control study	11/2009 02/2013	Endometriosis [1] stage III/IV (61) - 33 with OMA - 28 non-OMA/Tubal ligation [1] (33)	36.21 ± 8.37 * (Overall)	Complete blood cell count, NLR, PLR, and CA125 (before surgery [3])	No
Avcioğlu et al., 2014 [26]	Turkey	Retrospective study	01/2001 06/2013	Endometriosi [1] stage III/IV (124)/Endometriosis [1] stage I/II (40)	33.7 ± 7.7 * (Overall)	Complete blood cell count, MPV, PDW, and PCT (before surgery [3])	No
Kim et al., 2014 [27]	South Korea	Retrospective study	04/2005 03/2013	Endometriosis [1] stage III (189)/Endometriosis [1] stage IV (230)	15-51 (Overall) 19-49 - 33.8 ± 6.8 * (stage III) 15-51 - 34.7 ± 7.0 * (stage IV)	Complete blood cell count, NLR, CRP, AMH, CEA, CA125, CA 19-9 (<1 month before surgery)	No
Chmaj-Wierzchowska et al., 2015 [13]	Poland	Hospital-based case-control	09/2009 11/2012	OMA [1] without coexisting foci of peritoneal endometriosis (48)/Mature teratomas [1] (38)	18-38 (Overall) 30.00 ± 4.6 * (OMA) 27.03 ± 4.52 * (teratomas)	Complete blood cell count, fibrinogen, urocortin, ghrelin, and leptin (<1 day before surgery)	No
Yang et al., 2015 [24]	China	Retrospective case-control study	01/2009 06/2012 [4]	Endometriosis [1] - 119 Stage III - 78 Stage IV/ Benign ovarian cysts [1] (102) Healthy women [2] (112)	32.58 ± 6.37 * (Overall) 32.17 ± 6.50 * (endometriosis) 32.03 ± 6.83 * (benign ovarian cyst) 33.81 ± 5.52 * (healthy women)	Complete blood cell count, PLR, and CA125 (before surgery or as part of routine health examination [3])	Unclear
Wu et al., 2015 [12]	China	Hospital-based case-control	06-12/2012	OMA [1] (50) -35 stage III -15 stage IV/Age-matched healthy women [2] (50)	23-44 - 32.9 ± 6.1 * (OMA) 20-48 - 31.4 ± 6.4 * (controls)	Complete blood cell count, aPTT, PT, TT, INR, fibrinogen, D-dimer, fasting serum glucose, and serum cortisol (before surgery [3])	Yes

Table 5. Cont.

Author, Years	Country	Study Design	Study Period	Cases/Controls Sample Size (n)	Age (Years)	Parameters Assessed (When)	Confounding Factors
Tokmak et al., 2016 [9]	Turkey	Retrospective case-control study	01/2008 01/2013	OMA [1](467/Age- and BMI-matched benign ovarian cysts [1] (340)	16–50 (Overall) 18–49 −33.7 ± 8.4 * (OMA) 16–50 − 33.9 ± 11.6 * (Controls)	Complete blood cell count, NLR, PLR, CA125, AFP, CA 19-9, CA-15.3 (<1 month before surgery)	Unclear
Ding et al., 2018 [14]	China	Cross-sectional study	04/2015 03/2016	OMA [1] (100)/ Women without endometriosis (100): - 60 Healthy women [2] - 40 CIN III or ovarian teratoma [1]	21–49 (Overall) 32.0 ± 7.1 * (OMA) 33.0 ± 7.1 * (controls)	PLC, platelet activation rate, maximum platelet aggregation rate, D-dimer, fibrinogen, FDPs, sP-sel, F1 + 2, PT; TT; aPTT, INR (before surgery [3] and 3 months later only in OMA)	Unclear
Seckin et al., 2018 [28]	Turkey	Retrospective case-control study	01/2013 12/2016	OMA [1] (267)/ Benign ovarian cysts [1] (235)	15–49 − 27.1 ± 7.2 * (overall) 28.3 ± 6.6 * (cases) 25.8 ± 7.6 * (controls)	Complete blood cell count, NLR, PCT, PDW, PLR, and CA125 (before surgery [3])	Yes (only age </> 25 years)
Viganò et al., 2018 [14]	Italy	Retrospective case-control study	01/2013 12/2015	Endometriosis [1] (169) - 45 Stage I-II - 124 Stage III-IV/ Benign gynecologic pathology [1] (145)	35.8 ± 5.9 * (endometriosis) 36.9 ± 6.5 * (controls)	Complete blood cell count, NLR, PLR, TT ratio, aPTT, and INR (<1 month before surgery)	Yes
Coskun et al., 2019 [32]	Turkey	Retrospective case-control study	01/2013 01/2015	Adenomyosis [1] (84) Endometriosis [1] (102)/ Tubal ligation [1] (88)	52.9 ±7.4 * (adenomyosis) 35.3 ± 8.7 * (OMA) 37.9 ± 4.2 * (Controls)	Complete blood cell count, MPV, and CA125 (<1 week before the surgery)	Unclear
Ding et al., 2019 [30]	China	Retrospective case-control study	06/2015 06/2017	OMA [1] (226)/ Cyst group [1] (210) Tubal reanastomosis [1] (112)	35.7 ± 0.4 * (OMA) 35.9 ± 0.4 * (Cyst group) 35.8 ± 0.5 * (Controls)	Complete blood cell count, TT, PT, fibrinogen, CRP, PLR, NLR, aPTT, and CA125 (<1 month before surgery)	Yes
Turgut et al., 2019 [31]	Turkey	Retrospective case-control study	01/2012 02/2017	Endometriosis [1] (121) - 17 Stage I-II - 104 Stage III-IV Healthy women [2] (136)	22–53 (endometriosis) 17–51 (controls)	Complete blood cell count, MPV, and CA125 (before surgery [3])	Yes (age)

Note: * Mean ± SD. [1] Women with surgical and pathological diagnosis of endometriosis or other benign diseases/conditions with exclusion of endometriosis; [2] no surgery performed; [3] not specified when; [4] healthy women recruited only between 1/2012 and 06/2012; OMA, ovarian endometriosis; NLR, neutrophil–lymphocyte ratio; CA125, cancer antigen 125; PLR, platelet–lymphocyte ratio; MPV, mean platelet volume; PDW, platelet distribution width; PCT, plateletcrit; CPR, C-reactive protein; AMH, anti-Müllerian hormone; CEA, carcinoembryonic antigen; CA19-9, cancer antigen 19-9; aPTT, activated partial thromboplastin time; PT, prothrombin time; TT, thrombin time; INR, international normalized ratio; AFP, α-fetoprotein; CA15-3, cancer antigen 15-3; PLC, platelets; FDPs, fibrin degradation products; sP-sel, plasma-soluble P-selectin; F1 + 2, prothrombin fragment F1 + 2.

3.2.1. Coagulation Parameters in Endometriosis Patients

Table 6 shows the results of the studies that have investigated coagulation parameters in relation to the presence of endometriosis. The first studies that evaluated PLC did not find significant differences between endometriosis patients and the control groups [24,25]. The same results were obtained in other studies addressing PLC as a secondary outcome in the investigations of other coagulation parameters useful for the diagnosis of endometriosis [9,12–14,31]. In a retrospective case–control study that included women with adenomyosis, endometriosis, and a control group, Coskun et al. found a statistically higher PLC in endometriosis patients versus controls [32]. Similar results were obtained by Seckin and coworkers that, considering women with OMAs or other benign adnexal cysts, reported a significantly higher PLC in the OMA group compared to controls, and this difference remained even when considering the younger (<25 years old) and older (>25 years old) subgroups [28]. Avcioğlu et al. found that in patients with advanced endometriosis (stages III–IV), PLC was significantly higher when compared to minimal–mild endometriosis (stages I–II) and showed a significant positive correlation between PLC ($r = 0.8$; $p = 0.001$) and white blood cell (WBC) [26]. This finding was later supported by Ding et al., who reported a significantly higher PLC in women with endometriosis compared to controls and, within the OMA group, a significantly higher PLC mean value in case of severe endometriosis [30]. Opposite results were obtained by Kim and coworkers, since PLC was not significantly different in severe endometriosis [27]. Three studies have evaluated PT [12,29,30], and only Ding and coworkers showed a significantly shorter time in the OMA group compared to a benign cyst group and a control group [30]. Conversely, for TT, three studies [12,29,30] out of four showed significantly shorter values in patients affected by OMAs compared to control groups [12,14,29,30]. Three studies have evaluated differences in INR between patients with and without endometriosis finding no difference [12,14,29]. Four studies have addressed aPTT [12,14,29,30], and two of them have reported shortened aPTT in cases when compared to controls [12,14]. In particular, in our previous study, considering the various manifestations of endometriosis separately, we found that women with ovarian disease had shortened aPTT values in comparison to controls and women with SPE and DIE. In addition, women with stage I to II endometriosis had slightly shorter, but significant, aPTT values than those with stage III to IV disease [14]. In a multivariate logistic regression analysis, after controlling for potential confounders (age, parity, BMI, and smoking), aPTT retained significant predictive value for endometriosis [14]. Interestingly, in a cross-sectional study considering 100 women with OMA before and three months after surgery, Ding and colleagues found that, after the surgical removal of all visible lesions by laparoscopy, the coagulation measurements (PLC, INR, PT, aPTT, and TT) were all significantly changed suggesting a possible role for active endometriotic lesions in this modification [29].

Table 6. Systematic review: coagulation parameters of women with and without endometriosis in the included studies.

Author	Year	Study Population (n)	PT	TT	aPTT	PLC (10^9/L)	INR
Yavuzcan et al. [25]	2013	Cases (OMA): 33				269.8 ± 65.2	
		Cases (non-OMA): 28				298.9 ± 107.8	
		Controls: 33				286.4 ± 67.6	
Avcioğlu et al. [26]	2014	Stage I–II: 40				187 ± 36.18 *	
		Stage III–IV: 124				309.15 ± 54.43 *	
Kim et al. [27]	2014	Stage III (OMA): 189				NR	
		Stage IV (OMA): 230				NR	
Wu et al. [12]	2015	Cases (OMA): 50	NR	NR *	NR *	NR	NR
		Controls: 50	NR	NR *	NR *	NR	NR
Chmaj-Wierzchowska et al. [13]	2015	Cases (OMA): 48				267.80	
		Controls: 38				258.90	
Yang et al. [24]	2015	Cases: 197				253.25 ± 59.98	
		Benign tumor: 102				248.83 ± 61.69	
		Controls: 112				246.47 ± 52.55	
Tokmak et al. [9]	2016	Cases (OMA): 467				275.9 ± 72.1	
		Controls: 340				276.2 ± 71.3	
Seckin et al. [28]	2018	Cases (OMA): 267				292.9 ± 67.6 *	
		Controls: 235				269.7 ± 61.3 *	
		Cases: 169		1.00 ± 0.9	1.12 ± 0.19 *	250.00 ± 55.8	0.99 ± 056
Viganò et al. [14]	2018	Controls: 145		0.970 ± 0.10	1.13 ± 0.15 *	262.20 ± 63.4	0.98 ± 0.16
		Cases (OMA): 98		0.99 ± 0.06	1.08 ± 0.07 *	254.5 ± 61.47	0.99 ± 0.71
		Controls: 145		0.99 ± 0.09	1.14 ± 0.07 *	254.7 ± 58.62	0.99 ± 0.11
Ding et al. [29]	2018	Cases (OMA): 100	NR	NR *	NR	NR	NR
		Post-surgery (OMA): 100	NR	NR *	NR	NR	NR
		Cases: 121	NR *	NR *	NR *	NR *	NR *
Turgut et al. [31]	2019	Controls: 136				265 ± 86	
		Cases (OMA): 226	12.69 ± 0.04 *	15.42 ± 0.04 *	NR	258 ± 70.5	
		Controls: 112	12.99 ± 0.06 *	15.78 ± 0.06 *	NR	239.8 ± 3.6 *	
		Benign cyst: 210	13.00 ± 0.04 *	15.68 ± 0.05 *	NR	220.0 ± 5.4 *	
Ding et al. [30]	2019	Stage III (OMA): 91	12.64 ± 0.06	15.38 ± 0.06	35.68 ± 0.30	228.4 ± 4.0 *	
		Stage IV (OMA): 135	12.72 ± 0.05	15.44 ± 0.05	35.44 ± 0.26	243.8 ± 5.4 *	
		Cases: 102				237.1 ± 4.7 *	
Coskun et al. [32]	2019	Adenomyosis: 84				292.9 ± 73.9 *	
		Controls: 88				295.1 ± 77.5	
						269.9 ± 59 *	

Note: * statistically significant; PT: prothrombin time; TT: thrombin time; aPTT: activated partial thromboplastin time; PLC: platelet count; INR: international normalized ratio; OMA: ovarian endometrioma; NR: not reported.

3.2.2. Systemic Inflammatory Markers in Endometriosis Patients

Results for the inflammatory markers, including neutrophils, lymphocytes, PLR, and NLR, from the systematic review are presented in Table 7. Three studies showed that neutrophil count was higher in patients with endometriosis than in women without the disease [9,23,31]. On the other hand, three studies showed no significant difference among groups, either when considering OMAs or in non-OMA patients [14,25,28]. Importantly, our present study confirmed a significantly higher neutrophil count in patients with endometriosis. Among eight studies investigating the lymphocyte count [9,14,23–25,27,28,31], only three of them reported a significantly lower mean cell count in endometriosis compared to controls [9,23,31], and no correlation between the stage of endometriosis and the lymphocyte count was observed by Kim et al. [27]. Two studies found no difference between cases and controls in terms of NLR [25,28]. In our previous study, we found no difference in NLR between women with endometriosis and controls, although, when considering the various manifestations of endometriosis separately, a significant difference among groups emerged, as women with peritoneal lesions had lower NLR compared to patients without this form [14]. On the contrary, NLR was found to be significantly increased in the endometriosis group by Cho et al., who evaluated the usefulness of NLR in diagnosing endometriosis compared to benign ovarian tumors and healthy controls [23]. The same result was subsequently confirmed by three other studies [9,30,31]. Kim and coworkers, comparing stage I–II to stage III–IV endometriosis cases who underwent laparoscopic conservative surgery for OMAs, did not find any difference in NLR [27]. Among six studies investigating PLR [9,14,24,25,28,30], results obtained were more consistent. Four groups reported a significantly higher PLR in women with endometriosis [9,24,28,30]. In our previous case–control study [14], considering the various manifestations of endometriosis separately, we found that women with stage I to II endometriosis had significantly higher PLR than those with stage III to IV disease. A higher PLR in stage III–IV of endometriosis has been reported by Yang et al., compared to benign adnexal tumors and controls [24]. Only the study by Yavuzcan et al. reported no statistically significant difference in terms of PLR between endometriosis patients and controls and among the various endometriosis subgroups [25].

Table 7. Systematic review: inflammatory parameters of women with or without endometriosis in the included studies.

Author	Year	Study Population (n)	Neutrophils 10^9/L	Lymphocytes 10^9/L	NLR	PLR
Cho et al. [23]	2008	Cases: 231	4.41 *	1.82 *	2.66 *	
		Benign tumor: 145	4.17 *	1.96 *	2.31 *	
		Controls: 384	3.6 *	1.95 *	1.99 *	
Yavuzcan et al. [25]	2013	Cases (OMA): 33	4.14 ± 1.73	2.12 ± 0.87	2.40 ± 2.04	162.84 ± 141.28
		Cases (non-OMA): 28	4.68 ± 2.18	2.02 ± 0.68	2.51 ± 1.37	159.14 ± 61.20
		Controls:33	4.50 ± 1.57	2.25 ± 0.66	2.11 ± 0.86	132.45 ± 35.74
Kim et al. [27]	2014	Stage III (OMA): 189		NR	NR	
		Stage IV (OMA):230		NR	NR	
Yang et al. [24]	2015	Cases: 197		1.91 ± 0.52		141.79 ± 51.78 *
		Benign tumor:102		2.02 ± 0.52		129.28 ± 39.20 *
		Controls: 112		2.05 ± 0.49		126.68 ± 39.67 *
Tokmak et al. [9]	2016	Cases (OMA): 467	4.8 ± 1.8 *	1.98 ± 5.92 *	2.8 ± 2.0 *	153.3 ± 71.3 *
		Controls: 340	3.8 ± 1.2 *	2.41 ± 7.17 *	1.7 ± 0.5 *	122.4 ± 42.7 *
		Cases: 169	3.76 ± 1.34	2.04 ± 0.56	NR	NR
Viganò et al. [14]	2018	Cases (OMA): 98	3.9 ± 1.62	2.02 ± 0.66	2.08 ± 1.01	135.18 ± 68.69
		Controls:145	3.99 ± 1.6	1.97 ± 0.55	2.16 ± 1.25	130.65 ± 52.8
Seckin et al. [28]	2018	Cases: 267	4.6 ± 1.8	2.2 ± 0.6	2.3 ± 1.3	142.3 ± 48.4 *
		Controls:235	4.5 ± 2.1	2.2 ± 0.7	2.1 ± 1.2	129.3 ± 40.4 *
Turgut et al. [31]	2019	Cases: 121	4.4 ± 1.9 *	2 ± 0.8 *	2.18 ± 0.86 *	
		Controls:136	3.55 ± 1.53 *	2.15 ± 0.8 *	1.70 ± 0.8 *	
Ding et al. [30]	2019	Cases: 226 (OMA)			2.56 ± 0.07 *	146.4 ± 2.8 *
		Benign cyst: 210			2.34 ± 0.07 *	137.7 ± 3.4 *

Note: * p-value statistically significant; OMA: ovarian endometrioma; NLR: neutrophil-to-lymphocyte ratio; PLR: platelet-to-lymphocyte ratio; NR: not reported.

4. Discussion

We have herein confirmed our previous results documenting the present of subtle alterations of the peripheral coagulation system in patients with endometriosis. More specifically, in the validation study, the sub-analysis according to the various forms of the disease showed a shortened aPTT to be associated with the presence of moderate–severe endometriosis and with the presence of OMAs. This result is in line with previous evidence demonstrating a shortened aPTT in women with endometriosis, in particular with the ovarian form [12,14].

Results from the systematic reviews are characterized by a high variability, but a certain rate of consistency has been found also for alterations in TT and PLR in association with endometriosis.

In relation to the inflammatory parameters, we found a significantly higher neutrophil count in patients with endometriosis and a significantly lower absolute lymphocyte count in women affected by OMAs. We failed to detect similar results in our previous study thus supporting again the high variability of the observations. On the other hand, in line with our present findings, some groups had already reported that neutrophil count and NLR were significantly increased in the endometriosis group [9,23,30,31].

Variability of the results among the different studies may have different explanations. First, numbers of cases enrolled in the various studies are limited and, given the small changes observed among groups, the possibility of detecting significant differences is reduced. This is the reason for our choice to proceed with a systematic review. Second, the control groups are quite different among the studies, from only surgical patients as controls, or comparing women with other benign ovarian disease to endometriosis. A benign ovarian cyst may be responsible of an inflammatory pelvic environment as well, with a consequential alteration in inflammatory markers. Third, endometriosis is characterized by a plethora of manifestations and forms that are differently represented in the selected studies; some authors considered both minimal–mild and moderate–severe endometriosis, while other studies included only women with an advanced disease (stages III–IV) [27,30]. Similarly, some studies included only women without an ovarian disease while others considered only OMA patients [9,27,30] and others a combination of the two forms [25].

Overall, these results tend to confirm the idea that women with endometriosis are characterized by systemic changes of some inflammatory parameters [1,20,33,34] as well as by a modest change of the coagulation function. Indeed, all the modifications of the coagulation process detected are still within the normal reference intervals. Interestingly, Ding and coworkers have shown that three months after surgery for the removal of endometriotic lesions, the coagulation measurements were all significantly changed, suggesting a possible role for active endometriosis in the alterations of coagulation parameters, either locally or systemically [29].

The subtle variations observed in affected patients may be due to the TF pathway activation at the level of endometriotic lesions. Immunohistochemical studies revealed a marked elevation of TF expression pattern in eutopic and ectopic endometrium from women with endometriosis [35]. Moreover, the protease-activated receptor 2 (PAR-2), which is activated by TF/FVIIa, was as well demonstrated to be highly upregulated in the glandular epithelium of eutopic endometrium. Hence, both TF and the PAR-2 receptor are strategically poised for angiogenic and inflammatory signaling in endometriotic lesions [36,37]. Once TF is exposed to blood, it starts a reaction cascade that culminates in the increased production of thrombin. A shortened aPTT is correlated with elevated levels of coagulation factors (except factor VII) and of all markers for increased thrombin generation in plasma (prothrombin fragment 1,2, thrombin–antithrombin complexes, D-dimers, and factor VIII coagulant activity), thus determining a change in hemostatic balance in favor of a prothrombotic state [38,39]. In our multivariate logistic regression analysis, aPTT retained significant predictive value for stage III–IV endometriosis, but given the small difference detected, this diagnostic parameter is unlikely to be useful to fully differentiate women with and without disease. Endometriosis would not more frequently develop in women with shorter aPTT; however, we cannot exclude that these perturbations of the coagulation system may occur at some time during the pathogenetic process starting from repeated tissue repair lesions. Indeed, cyclic bleeding of endometriotic lesions determines the local release of factors such as those activating platelets (PAFs), thrombin and thromboxane A2 (TXA2), resulting in increased angiogenesis, increased vascular permeability and in the induction of platelet activation and aggregation [4,40–42]. The activated platelets would further release von Willebrand factor (vWF), adenosine diphosphate (ADP), serotonin, PAF, TXA2, and Chemokine (C-X-C motif) ligand 4 (CXCL4), causing further platelet aggregation and perpetuating the coagulation activation [43]. Importantly, the consequent extravasation and aggregation of platelets can finally induce fibrosis in endometriosis lesions through TGF-β1 release and induction of the TGF-β1/Smad3 signaling pathway, which is a potent inducer of epithelial–mesenchymal transition and fibroblast-to-myofibroblast transition in endometriotic cells [40,43,44].

Controversial data have been reported in relation to the platelet count among the various studies, while a quite consistent significantly higher PLR was observed in women in endometriosis. A possible explanation for this inconsistency is that platelets exert their role as "activated platelets", without necessarily increasing their absolute mean value in peripheral blood. The elevated percentage of activated platelets in the peripheral blood of women with endometriosis is consistent with the observed shortened TT and aPTT. The release of TXA2, a potent platelet activation inducer, can generate a vicious cycle in maintaining platelet activation, the activation of the coagulation cascade, higher plasma fibrinogen levels, and short aPTTs in endometriosis [44,45].

Recently, increased cardiovascular and thrombotic morbidity in terms of myocardial infarction, angina, and coronary bypass graft intervention has been recognized in women with endometriosis. The relative risk of combined coronary heart disease events was 1.62 (95% confidence interval: 1.39–1.89) after adjustment for confounders [46,47]. Moreover, endometriosis has been interestingly identified as a novel predicting factor for venous thromboembolism during pregnancy and postpartum in a Japanese birth cohort study [48]. Factors contributing to this increased risk have not been deeply investigated. Possible causes could be the hormonal treatment or previous hysterectomy/oophorectomy in affected women. On the other hand, another hypothesis could attribute these events to these subtle alterations in coagulation and fibrinolysis parameters recently identified in affected patients causing a hypercoagulable status [12].

Our validation study has some limitations: (1) the retrospective design of the study that could have influenced the interpretation of the data; (2) patients on hormonal treatment have been included, but, in order to evaluate the unique effect of the endometriosis on the coagulation status, we did include only cases and controls with a negative history of hormonal therapy before surgery in the comparisons of coagulation parameters; (3) age was different between cases and controls; nevertheless, since a limited age range was set as a case selection criteria, a selection bias may be excluded.

5. Conclusions

In conclusion, our findings suggest that women with OMAs and moderate–severe forms of endometriosis show a modest strength of the coagulation function potentially attributable to the inflammatory nature of the lesions. Endometriosis also seems to be associated with systemic changes of some inflammatory parameters, for instance, a modest increase of neutrophil count. All the alterations detected are still within the normal reference intervals, explaining the high heterogeneity among studies. We cannot, however, rule out that these systemic perturbations may contribute to the pathogenetic process of the disease or to the increased cardiovascular and thrombotic morbidity observed in patients affected.

Supplementary Materials: The following are available online at http://www.mdpi.com/2075-4418/10/8/567/s1, Figure S1: Risk-of-bias assessment.

Author Contributions: Conceptualization, P.V. and J.O.; methodology, P.V.; software, N.S.; validation, P.V., M.C., and J.O.; formal analysis, N.S.; investigation, M.S., L.B., and R.V.; resources, M.S., L.B., R.V., N.S., and C.D.; data curation, N.S. and J.O.; writing—original draft preparation, M.S., L.B., N.S., R.V., C.D., and P.V.; writing—review and editing, J.O. and P.V.; visualization, J.O., P.V., and M.C.; supervision, J.O., P.V., and M.C.; project administration, M.C. and P.V. All authors have read and agreed to the published version of the manuscript.

Funding: This research received no external funding.

Conflicts of Interest: The authors declare no conflict of interest in relation to this study.

References

1. Vercellini, P.P.; Vigano, P.; Somigliana, E.; Fedele, L. Endometriosis: Pathogenesis and treatment. *Nat. Rev. Endocrinol.* **2013**, *10*, 261–275. [CrossRef]
2. Zondervan, K.; Becker, C.M.; Koga, K.; Missmer, S.A.; Taylor, R.N.; Vigano, P. Endometriosis. *Nat. Rev. Dis. Prim.* **2018**, *4*, 9. [CrossRef]
3. Vigano, P.; Candiani, M.; Monno, A.; Giacomini, E.; Vercellini, P.P.; Somigliana, E. Time to redefine endometriosis including its pro-fibrotic nature. *Hum. Reprod.* **2018**, *33*, 347–352. [CrossRef]
4. Vigano, P.; Ottolina, J.; Bartiromo, L.; Bonavina, G.; Schimberni, M.; Villanacci, R.; Candiani, M. Cellular Components Contributing to Fibrosis in Endometriosis: A Literature Review. *J. Minim. Invasive Gynecol.* **2020**, *27*, 287–295. [CrossRef]
5. Sikora, J.; Mielczarek-Palacz, A.; Kondera-Anasz, Z. Imbalance in Cytokines from Interleukin-1 Family - Role in Pathogenesis of Endometriosis. *Am. J. Reprod. Immunol.* **2012**, *68*, 138–145. [CrossRef]
6. Wickiewicz, D.; Chrobak, A.; Gmyrek, G.B.; Halbersztadt, A.; Gabryś, M.; Goluda, M.; Chełmońska-Soyta, A. Diagnostic accuracy of interleukin-6 levels in peritoneal fluid for detection of endometriosis. *Arch. Gynecol. Obstet.* **2013**, *288*, 805–814. [CrossRef]
7. Birt, J.A.; Nabli, H.; Stilley, J.A.; Windham, E.A.; Frazier, S.R.; Sharpe-Timms, K.L. Elevated Peritoneal Fluid TNF-α Incites Ovarian Early Growth Response Factor 1 Expression and Downstream Protease Mediators. *Reprod. Sci.* **2013**, *20*, 514–523. [CrossRef] [PubMed]
8. Velasco, I.; Acién, P.; Campos, A.; Acién, M.I.; Ruiz-Maciá, E. Interleukin-6 and other soluble factors in peritoneal fluid and endometriomas and their relation to pain and aromatase expression. *J. Reprod. Immunol.* **2010**, *84*, 199–205. [CrossRef] [PubMed]
9. Tokmak, A.; Yildirim, G.; Öztaş, E.; Akar, S.; Erkenekli, K.; Gülşen, P.; Yilmaz, N.; Uğur, M. Use of Neutrophil-to-Lymphocyte Ratio Combined With CA-125 to Distinguish Endometriomas From Other Benign Ovarian Cysts. *Reprod. Sci.* **2015**, *23*, 795–802. [CrossRef] [PubMed]
10. Boss, E.A.; Massuger, L.F.A.G.; Thomas, C.M.; Geurts-Moespot, A.; Van Schaik, J.H.M.; Boonstra, H.; Sweep, F.C.G.J. Clinical value of components of the plasminogen activation system in ovarian cyst fluid. *Anticancer. Res.* **2002**, *22*, 275–282.
11. Esmon, C.T. The interactions between inflammation and coagulation. *Br. J. Haematol.* **2005**, *131*, 417–430. [CrossRef] [PubMed]
12. Wu, Q.; Ding, D.; Liu, X.; Guo, S.-W. Evidence for a Hypercoagulable State in Women With Ovarian Endometriomas. *Reprod. Sci.* **2015**, *22*, 1107–1114. [CrossRef] [PubMed]
13. Chmaj-Wierzchowska, K.; Kampioni, M.; Wilczak, M.; Sajdak, S.; Opala, T. Novel markers in the diagnostics of endometriosis: Urocortin, ghrelin, and leptin or leukocytes, fibrinogen, and CA-125? *Taiwan. J. Obstet. Gynecol.* **2015**, *54*, 126–130. [CrossRef] [PubMed]
14. Also, P.; Ottolina, J.; Sarais, V.; Rebonato, G.; Somigliana, E.; Candiani, M. Coagulation Status in Women With Endometriosis. *Reprod. Sci.* **2017**, *25*, 559–565. [CrossRef]
15. Sanchez, A.M.; Vigano, P.; Somigliana, E.; Panina-Bordignon, P.; Vercellini, P.P.; Candiani, M. The distinguishing cellular and molecular features of the endometriotic ovarian cyst: From pathophysiology to the potential endometrioma-mediated damage to the ovary. *Hum. Reprod. Updat.* **2013**, *20*, 217–230. [CrossRef]
16. Reproductive, A.S.F. Revised American Society for Reproductive Medicine classification of endometriosis: 1996. *Fertil. Steril.* **1997**, *67*, 817–821. [CrossRef]
17. Nisolle, M.; Donnez, J. Peritoneal endometriosis, ovarian endometriosis, and adenomyotic nodules of the rectovaginal septum are three different entities. *Fertil. Steril.* **1997**, *68*, 585–596. [CrossRef]

18. Moher, D.; Liberati, A.; Tetzlaff, J.; Altman, D.G. Preferred Reporting Items for Systematic Reviews and Meta-Analyses: The PRISMA Statement. *Ann. Intern. Med.* **2009**, *151*, 264–269. [CrossRef]
19. EFSA Scientific Committee; Benford, D.; Halldorsson, T.; Jeger, M.J.; Knutsen, H.K.; More, S.; Naegeli, H.; Noteborn, H.; Ockleford, C.; Ricci, A.; et al. The principles and methods behind EFSA's Guidance on Uncertainty Analysis in Scientific Assessment. *EFSA J.* **2018**, *16*, 5122. [CrossRef]
20. Vigano, P.; Somigliana, E.; Panina, P.; Rabellotti, E.; Vercellini, P.P.; Candiani, M. Principles of phenomics in endometriosis. *Hum. Reprod. Updat.* **2012**, *18*, 248–259. [CrossRef]
21. World Health Organization Collaborative Study of Cardiovascular Disease and Steroid Hormone Contarception Venous thromboembolic disease and combined oral contraceptives: Results of international multicentre case-control study. *Lancet* **1995**, *346*, 1575–1582. [CrossRef]
22. Farmer, R.; Lawrenson, R.; Thompson, C.; Kennedy, J.; Hambleton, I.R. Population-based study of risk of venous thromboembolism associated with various oral contraceptives. *Lancet* **1997**, *349*, 83–88. [CrossRef]
23. Cho, S.; Cho, H.; Nam, A.; Kim, H.Y.; Choi, Y.S.; Park, K.H.; Cho, D.J.; Lee, B.S. Neutrophil-to-lymphocyte ratio as an adjunct to CA-125 for the diagnosis of endometriosis. *Fertil. Steril.* **2008**, *90*, 2073–2079. [CrossRef]
24. Yang, H.; Zhu, L.; Wang, S.; Lang, J.; Xu, T. Noninvasive Diagnosis of Moderate to Severe Endometriosis: The Platelet-Lymphocyte Ratio Cannot Be a Neoadjuvant Biomarker for Serum Cancer Antigen 125. *J. Minim. Invasive Gynecol.* **2015**, *22*, 373–377. [CrossRef] [PubMed]
25. Yavuzcan, A.; Caglar, M.; Ustun, Y.; Dilbaz, S.; Ozdemir, I.; Yıldız, E.; Ozkara, A.; Kumru, S. Evaluation of mean platelet volume, neutrophil/lymphocyte ratio and platelet/lymphocyte ratio in advanced stage endometriosis with endometrioma. *J. Turk. Gynecol. Assoc.* **2013**, *14*, 210–215. [CrossRef]
26. Avcioğlu, S.N.; Altinkaya, S.Ö.; Küçük, M.; Demircan-Sezer, S.; Yüksel, H. Can Platelet Indices Be New Biomarkers for Severe Endometriosis? *ISRN Obstet. Gynecol.* **2014**, *2014*, 1–6. [CrossRef]
27. Kim, S.K.; Park, J.Y.; Jee, B.C.; Suh, C.S.; Kim, S.H. Association of the neutrophil-to-lymphocyte ratio and CA 125 with the endometriosis score. *Clin. Exp. Reprod. Med.* **2014**, *41*, 151–157. [CrossRef]
28. Seckin, B.; Ates, M.C.; Kirbas, A.; Yesilyurt, H. Usefulness of hematological parameters for differential diagnosis of endometriomas in adolescents/young adults and older women. *Int. J. Adolesc. Med. Health* **2018**. [CrossRef]
29. Ding, D.; Liu, X.; Guo, S.-W. Further Evidence for Hypercoagulability in Women With Ovarian Endometriomas. *Reprod. Sci.* **2018**, *25*, 1540–1548. [CrossRef]
30. Ding, S.; Lin, Q.; Zhu, T.; Li, T.; Zhu, L.; Wang, J.; Zhang, X. Is there a correlation between inflammatory markers and coagulation parameters in women with advanced ovarian endometriosis? *BMC Women's Health* **2019**, *19*, 1–8. [CrossRef]
31. Turgut, A.; Hocaoglu, M.; Ozdamar, O.; Usta, A.; Gunay, T.; Akdeniz, E. Could hematologic parameters be useful biomarkers for the diagnosis of endometriosis? *Bratisl. Med. J.* **2019**, *120*, 912–918. [CrossRef] [PubMed]
32. Çoşkun, B.; Ince, O.; Erkilinc, S.; Elmas, B.; Saridogan, E.; Çoşkun, B.; Doğanay, M.; Erkılınç, S.; Saridogan, E. The feasibility of the platelet count and mean platelet volume as markers of endometriosis and adenomyosis: A case control study. *J. Gynecol. Obstet. Hum. Reprod.* **2019**, 101626. [CrossRef]
33. Cassarino, M.F.; Ambrogio, A.G.; Cassarino, A.; Terreni, M.R.; Gentilini, D.; Sesta, A.; Cavagnini, F.; Losa, M.; Giraldi, F.P. Gene expression profiling in human corticotroph tumours reveals distinct, neuroendocrine profiles. *J. Neuroendocr.* **2018**, *30*, e12628. [CrossRef] [PubMed]
34. Sanchez, A.M.; Somigliana, E.; Vercellini, P.; Pagliardini, L.; Candiani, M.; Viganò, P. Endometriosis as a detrimental condition for granulosa cell steroidogenesis and development: From molecular alterations to clinical impact. *J. Steroid Biochem. Mol. Biol.* **2016**, *155*, 35–46. [CrossRef] [PubMed]
35. Krikun, G.; Lockwood, C.J.; Paidas, M.J. Tissue factor and the endometrium: From physiology to pathology. *Thromb. Res.* **2009**, *124*, 393–396. [CrossRef] [PubMed]
36. Lin, M.; Weng, H.; Wang, X.; Zhou, B.; Yu, P.; Wang, Y. The role of tissue factor and protease-activated receptor 2 in endometriosis. *Am. J. Reprod. Immunol.* **2012**, *68*, 251–257. [CrossRef]
37. Osuga, Y. Proteinase-activated receptors in the endometrium and endometriosis. *Front. Biosci.* **2012**, *4*, 1201–1212. [CrossRef]
38. Senthil, M.; Chaudhary, P.; Smith, D.; Ventura, P.E.; Frankel, P.H.; Pullarkat, V.; Trisal, V. A shortened activated partial thromboplastin time predicts the risk of catheter-associated venous thrombosis in cancer patients. *Thromb. Res.* **2014**, *134*, 165–168. [CrossRef]

39. Mina, A.; Favaloro, E.J.; Koutts, J. Relationship between short activated partial thromboplastin times, thrombin generation, procoagulant factors and procoagulant phospholipid activity. *Blood Coagul. Fibrinolysis* **2012**, *23*, 203–207. [CrossRef]
40. Guo, S.-W.; Ding, D.; Geng, J.-G.; Wang, L.; Liu, X. P-selectin as a potential therapeutic target for endometriosis. *Fertil. Steril.* **2015**, *103*, 990–1000.e8. [CrossRef]
41. Zhang, Q.; Duan, J.; Olson, M.; Fazleabas, A.T.; Guo, S.-W. Cellular Changes Consistent With Epithelial–Mesenchymal Transition and Fibroblast-to-Myofibroblast Transdifferentiation in the Progression of Experimental Endometriosis in Baboons. *Reprod. Sci.* **2016**, *23*, 1409–1421. [CrossRef] [PubMed]
42. Zhang, Q.; Duan, J.; Liu, X.; Guo, S.-W. Platelets drive smooth muscle metaplasia and fibrogenesis in endometriosis through epithelial–mesenchymal transition and fibroblast-to-myofibroblast transdifferentiation. *Mol. Cell. Endocrinol.* **2016**, *428*, 1–16. [CrossRef] [PubMed]
43. Guo, S.-W.; Du, Y.; Liu, X. Endometriosis-Derived Stromal Cells Secrete Thrombin and Thromboxane A2, Inducing Platelet Activation. *Reprod. Sci.* **2016**, *23*, 1044–1052. [CrossRef] [PubMed]
44. Ding, D.; Liu, X.; Duan, J.; Guo, S.-W. Platelets are an unindicted culprit in the development of endometriosis: Clinical and experimental evidence. *Hum. Reprod.* **2015**, *30*, 812–832. [CrossRef] [PubMed]
45. Mikhailidis, D.P.; Barradas, M.A.; Maris, A.; Jeremy, J.Y.; Dandona, P. Fibrinogen mediated activation of platelet aggregation and thromboxane A2 release: Pathological implications in vascular disease. *J. Clin. Pathol.* **1985**, *38*, 1166–1171. [CrossRef]
46. Kvaskoff, M.; Mu, F.; Terry, K.L.; Harris, H.R.; Poole, E.M.; Farland, L.V.; Missmer, S.A. Endometriosis: A high-risk population for major chronic diseases? *Hum. Reprod. Updat.* **2015**, *21*, 500–516. [CrossRef]
47. Zuin, M.; Rigatelli, G.; Stellin, G.; Faggian, G.; Roncon, L. Should women with endometriosis be screened for coronary artery disease? *Eur. J. Intern. Med.* **2016**, *35*, e19–e20. [CrossRef]
48. Sugiura-Ogasawara, M.; Ebara, T.; Matsuki, T.; Yamada, Y.; Omori, T.; Matsumoto, Y.; Kato, S.; Kano, H.; Kurihara, T.; Saitoh, S.; et al. Endometriosis and Recurrent Pregnancy Loss as New Risk Factors for Venous Thromboembolism during Pregnancy and Post-Partum: The JECS Birth Cohort. *Thromb. Haemost.* **2019**, *119*, 606–617. [CrossRef]

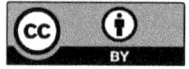

© 2020 by the authors. Licensee MDPI, Basel, Switzerland. This article is an open access article distributed under the terms and conditions of the Creative Commons Attribution (CC BY) license (http://creativecommons.org/licenses/by/4.0/).

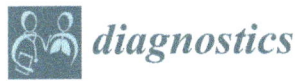

Article

BIRC5/Survivin Expression as a Non-Invasive Biomarker of Endometriosis

Carolina Filipchiuk [1], Antonio Simone Laganà [2,*], Rubia Beteli [3], Tatiana Guida Ponce [4], Denise Maria Christofolini [3], Camila Martins Trevisan [4], Fernando Luiz Affonso Fonseca [5], Caio Parente Barbosa [3] and Bianca Bianco [1,3]

1. Center of Natural and Human Sciences (CCNH), Universidade Federal do ABC, Santo André 09210-580, SP, Brazil; carol_f24@hotmail.com (C.F.); bianca.bianco@fmabc.br (B.B.)
2. Department of Obstetrics and Gynecology, "Filippo Del Ponte" Hospital, University of Insubria, 2100 Varese, Italy
3. Discipline of Sexual and Reproductive Health and Populational Genetics, Department of Collective Health, Faculdade de Medicina do ABC/Centro Universitário Saúde ABC, Santo André 09210-580, Brazil; rubs.fmabc@gmail.com (R.B.); denise.christofolini@fmabc.br (D.M.C.); caio.parente@fmabc.br (C.P.B.)
4. Postgraduate Program in Health Sciences, Faculdade de Medicina do ABC/Centro Universitário Saúde ABC, Santo André 09210-580, Brazil; tatianaguidaponce@gmail.com (T.G.P.); camilatrevisan22@gmail.com (C.M.T.)
5. Discipline of Clinical Analysis, Deparment of Patology, Faculdade de Medicina do ABC/Centro Universitário Saúde ABC, Santo André 09210-580, Brazil; profferfonseca@gmail.com
* Correspondence: antoniosimone.lagana@uninsubria.it

Received: 17 July 2020; Accepted: 28 July 2020; Published: 30 July 2020

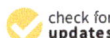

Abstract: The etiology of endometriosis is highly complex, and although it is a benign disease, it has several biological behaviors similar to malignant lesions, including cell invasion, neo-angiogenesis, and decreased apoptosis. Survivin is a protein encoded by the *BIRC5* gene that plays a role in cell division by inhibiting apoptosis and regulating the process of mitosis in embryonic and cancer cells. Therefore, we aimed to evaluate the expression of *BIRC5* in samples of peripheral blood of women with and without endometriosis. This study comprised of 40 women with endometriosis and 10 healthy women as controls. Peripheral blood samples were collected in the three phases of the menstrual cycle (follicular, ovulatory, and luteal). The expression of the *BIRC5* gene was evaluated by RT-qPCR using the TaqMan methodology. The *BIRC5* expression was significantly higher in all phases of the menstrual cycle in women with endometriosis, regardless of the disease stage. The accuracy of *BIRC5* expression in the peripheral blood for the diagnosis endometriosis presented AUC of 0.887 ($p < 0.001$), with 97.2% of sensitivity and specificity of 65.5% considering the overall endometriosis group. Regarding the minimal/mild endometriosis group, the AUC presented a value of 0.925 ($p < 0.001$), with 100% of sensitivity and 79.3% of specificity, whereas in the moderate/severe endometriosis group the AUC was 0.868 ($p < 0.001$), with a sensitivity of 95.8% and specificity of 65.5%. These findings suggest that the expression of *BIRC5* may be a potential noninvasive biomarker for the diagnosis of endometriosis.

Keywords: endometriosis; survivin; *BIRC5*; apoptosis; inhibitor of apoptosis protein

1. Introduction

Endometriosis is a common estrogen-dependent gynecological condition, which can affect women at a reproductive age [1]. It is defined as the presence of endometrial-like tissue outside of the uterus, often associated with chronic and inflammatory reaction [2]. The symptoms of endometriosis may vary from severe dysmenorrhea, dyspareunia, or chronic pelvic pain [1–3] to unexplained infertility, although the disease can be asymptomatic [4].

Cancer antigen 125 (CA125) plasma concentrations, a glycoprotein of epithelial origin, although largely used, are not reliable to diagnose endometriosis. Indeed, it may be elevated in several benign diseases and patients with non-ovarian malignancies, including cancers of the endometrium, lung, breast, pancreas, and colon [5], and it has no value in the diagnosis as a single test [3]. Indeed, according to guidelines of the European Society of Human Reproduction and Embryology (ESHRE), clinicians are recommended not to use immunological biomarkers, including CA125, in plasma, urine, or serum to diagnose endometriosis [6]. Despite considerable efforts towards searching for noninvasive diagnostic methods to detect endometriosis, the diagnosis can be suspected by ultrasound and/or other imaging methods [7] and confirmed only through laparoscopy with inspection of the abdominal cavity and histological confirmation of the lesion(s) [1,3]. As the surgery presents risks and also a high cost, a less invasive, but accurate test could lead to the diagnosis of the disease without the need for surgery, or at least it could help reduce the need for a surgical procedure for its confirmation [3].

The pathogenesis of endometriosis is still debated, although genetics, epigenetics, and immune elements may all play a pivotal role [8–10]. There are several theories to account for the origin of endometriosis and to explain how ectopic tissue can implant throughout the abdominal cavity [11]. However, there is no single theory that explains all of the different clinical presentations and pathological features in endometriosis [10]. A growing body of evidence has identified several comorbidities that are associated with endometriosis, including congenital uterine anomalies, autoimmune disease, allergy, cancers, and cardiovascular disease [12,13]. Melin et al. [14], based on 64,492 registers of the National Swedish Inpatient and Cancer Registrar data from 1969 to 2000, observed that women with endometriosis have an increased risk of some malignancies, particularly ovarian cancer. In addition, Wang et al. [15] in a recent meta-analysis comprising a total of 40,609 cases of epithelial ovarian cancer and 368,452 controls from 38 publications, also found that endometriosis was associated with an increased risk of epithelial ovarian cancer (OR = 1.42, 95% CI = 1.28–1.57). Endometriosis and cancer present similarities [16], such as cell invasion, unrestrained growth, neo-angiogenesis, and decreased apoptosis [17,18], although the first condition is clearly not neoplastic.

Inhibitors of apoptosis proteins (IAPs) have emerged as modulators in an evolutionarily conserved step in apoptosis, as negative regulatory proteins that prevent apoptotic cell death. Survivin, a member of the IAP family, is encoded by the *BIRC5* (baculoviral IAP repeat-containing 5) gene located at 17q25, and it plays a role in cell division by inhibiting apoptosis and regulating the process of mitosis in embryonic cells during embryogenesis and in cancer cells during tumorigenesis and tumor metastasis [19]. It also participates in chromosome division and segregation, proliferation, stress response, and angiogenesis [20]. In addition, survivin is considered a key element for the metastasis phenomenon [21–24] and, consequently, has received significant attention as a potential oncotherapeutic target [25].

Survivin expression in normal endometrium shows cyclic alterations dependent on the menstrual cycle [26–28]. In addition, survivin overexpression is shown to be present in hormone-dependent endometrial disorders, such as endometrial hyperplasia, carcinomas, and endometriosis [27–30]. Therefore, the aim of the present study was to evaluate the expression of *BIRC5* in samples of peripheral blood of women with and without endometriosis.

2. Materials and Methods

2.1. Participants

This case-control study was performed between February 2017 and December 2018 and comprised 50 women recruited at the Human Reproduction and Genetics Center of the Faculdade de Medicina do ABC, Santo Andre, Brazil. The design, analysis, interpretation of data, drafting, and revisions followed the Helsinki Declaration and the strengthening the reporting of observational studies in epidemiology (STROBE) statement, available through the enhancing the quality and transparency of health research (EQUATOR) network (www.equator-network.org). The study design was approved by the independent Research Ethics Committee of the "Faculdade de Medicina do ABC" (approve code

CAEE 64005816.8.0000.0082, approved on 1 February 2017). Each patient enrolled in this study signed an informed consent for all the procedures and to allow data and biological sample collection and analysis for research purposes. The study was non-advertised, and no remuneration was offered to encourage patients to give consent for the collection and analysis of their data. An independent data monitoring committee evaluated the interim and final data analysis of the study.

The endometriosis group comprised 40 women who had endometriosis diagnosed by laparoscopy and histological confirmation, classified according to the revised American Society for Reproductive Medicine (rASRM) score [31]. In this group, minimal/mild (stage I and II) endometriosis was found in 33.3% (12/36) of the cases, whereas moderate/severe (stage III and IV) endometriosis was found in 66.7% (24/36) of the cases. The surgical indication for all patients was infertility. The control group was carefully selected and comprised of 10 healthy and non-menopausal women who had no personal and/or familial history of endometriosis, autoimmune diseases, or cancer. All these women previously underwent tubal ligation for family planning reasons, and the absence of endometriosis was confirmed through inspection of the pelvic cavity.

2.2. Sample Collection

Fifteen milliliters of the peripheral blood samples were collected in a tube containing clot-separator gel and in a tube containing PAXgene Blood RNA (PreAnalytiX, BD Diagnostics®, Franklin Lakes, NJ, USA). After collection, the tubes for the biochemical dosages were centrifuged (1000 rpm for 10 min), the plasma was aliquoted into microtubes and frozen at −80 °C for further determination of follicle-stimulating hormone (FSH), luteinizing hormone (LH), progesterone, prolactin, and CA125 concentrations. The tube for RNA extraction was stored at −80 °C until extraction.

The samples for RNA extraction were collected in the three phases of the menstrual cycle (follicular, ovulatory, and luteal) for all women of the control group. Among the women of the endometriosis group, the samples were collected in 38.9% of women (14/36) in the follicular phase, 27.8% (10/36) in the ovulatory phase, and in 33.3% (12/36) in the luteal phase.

2.3. Hormonal Measurement

The hormonal profile was measured during the investigation into the cause of infertility. Progesterone and prolactin were measured at the luteal phase and FSH and LH at the follicular phase of the menstrual cycle. The hormones were measured by enzyme-linked fluorescent immunoassay (BioMerieux®, Hazelwood, MO, USA).

2.4. RT-qPCR

RNA extraction was carried out with Qiazol Lysis Reagent according to the manufacturer's instructions (Qiagen Inc., Valencia, CA, USA) and then total RNA was treated with DNase-I endonuclease (Thermo Fisher Scientific, Waltham, MA, USA). RNA sample concentrations were analyzed using a Nanodrop 2000 spectrophotometer (Thermo Fisher Scientific, Waltham, MA, USA) and the RNA integrity was analyzed via agarose gel electrophoresis to identify the 28S and 18S ribosomal rRNA. The cDNA synthesis was done with 1 μg of total RNA using a high capacity cDNA reverse transcription kit (Thermo Fisher Scientific, Waltham, MA, USA) following the manufacturer's guidelines.

The expression of *BIRC5* (Hs04194392_s1) and glyceraldehyde3-phosphate dehydrogenase (GAPDH, Hs99999905_m1) genes was measured by RT-qPCR, based on the TaqMan methodology (ThermoFisher Scientific, Waltham, MA, USA) using the equipment StepOne Real-Time PCR System (Applied Biosystems, Foster City, CA, USA). PCR reactions were processed to a final volume of 20 mL containing 10 μL of 2× TaqMan Universal PCR Master Mix, 1.25 μL TaqMan assay (20×), 2 μL of sample cDNA, and 6.75 μL of RNAse-free water. Reactions were performed at 95 °C for 10 min, followed by 40 cycles of 95 °C for 15 s, and annealing/extension at 60 °C for 60 s. Each reaction was performed in triplicates. The gene expression results were obtained using the $2^{-\Delta Ct}$.

2.5. Statistical Analyses

Statistical analyses were performed using GraphPad Software (v.7, LLC, San Diego, CA, USA, https://www.graphpad.com). Data normality was verified with the Shapiro–Wilk test. Variables were presented by medians with 95% confidence intervals (CI). Differences between two groups were tested by Mann–Whitney or Kruskal–Wallis tests. A Spearman's correlation test was performed to analyze the correlation between hormonal levels and the *BIRC5* expression. To test for accuracy, receiver operator characteristic (ROC) analysis was used and specificity, sensibility, predictive values, and 95% confidence interval (95% CI) were calculated. Statistical significance was considered when $p < 0.05$.

3. Results

Table 1 shows the comparison of clinical and hormonal characteristics of women with and without endometriosis. Hormonal values were in accordance with the reference values for each phase of the menstrual cycle. CA125, FSH, and prolactin levels were significantly higher in women with endometriosis compared with the control group. Conversely, age, body mass index (BMI), LH, and progesterone levels were not significantly different between groups. Regarding the endometriosis stage, all the parameters were not significantly different between women with minimal/mild and moderate/severe disease.

Figure 1A shows the comparison of *BIRC5* expression among women with endometriosis and according to the disease stage and the control group. The *BIRC5* expression was also significantly higher in women with endometriosis, regardless of the endometriosis stage (minimal/mild and moderate/severe endometriosis). Figure 1B shows the comparison of *BIRC5* expression between women with and without endometriosis in different phases of the menstrual cycle. The *BIRC5* expression was significantly higher in all phases of the menstrual cycle in women with endometriosis.

The correlation between hormonal levels and *BIRC5* expression in peripheral blood of women with endometriosis is reported in Table 2. Spearman's correlation coefficient showed that the progesterone was correlated with *BIRC5* expression (rho = 0.382, $p = 0.045$).

Table 1. Comparison of clinical and hormonal characteristics of women with and without endometriosis.

Variable *	Endometriosis ($n = 36$)	Controls ($n = 10$)	p **
Age (years)	35 (33.0–38.0)	33 (32–34.5)	0.933
BMI (kg/m^2)	24.3 (23.1–25.4)	24.7 (23.8–25.7)	0.800
CA125 (mUI/mL)	49.8 (22.6–67.6)	18.9 (15.2–36.3)	<0.001
FSH (mUI/mL)	7.2 (6.8–8.2)	6.4 (6.1–6.9)	<0.001
LH (mUI/mL)	6.3 (4.3–8.3)	6.7 (5.0–8.3)	0.838
Progesterone (ng/mL)	8.9 (6.9–11.0)	5.9 (2.9–8.9)	0.061
Prolactin (ng/mL)	17.1 (11.9–22.6)	8.5 (6.5–15.1)	0.010

* Median and 95% confidence interval. BMI, body mass index; CA125, cancer antigen 125; FSH, follicle-stimulating hormone; LH, luteinizing hormone. ** Mann–Whitney test.

Table 2. Correlation between hormone levels and *BICR5* expression in peripheral blood of women with endometriosis.

	rho *	p
CA125	−0.191	0.265
FSH	0.276	0.115
LH	0.274	0.117
Progesterone	0.382	0.045
Prolactin	−0.030	0.873

* Spearman's correlation. CA125, cancer antigen 125; FSH, follicle-stimulating hormone; LH, luteinizing hormone.

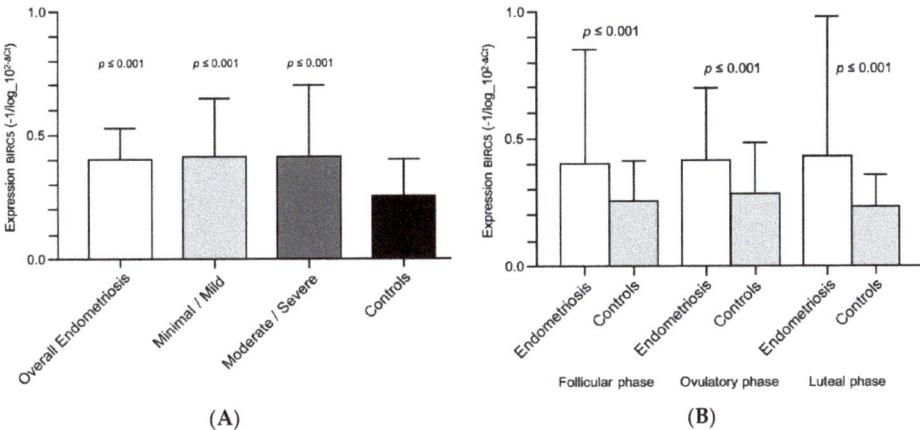

Figure 1. (**A**) *BIRC5* expression in the peripheral blood samples of women with endometriosis according to the disease stage. (**B**) *BIRC5* expression in the peripheral blood samples of women with and without endometriosis in different phases of the menstrual cycle.

To estimate the accuracy of *BIRC5* expression in the peripheral blood to diagnostic endometriosis and also according to disease staging, the area under the ROC curve was analyzed (Figure 2).

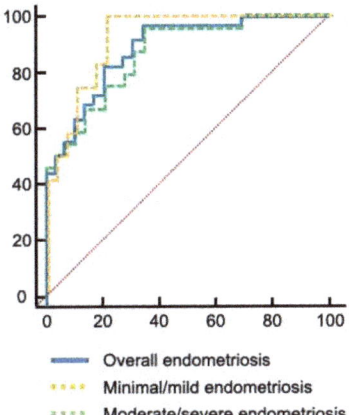

Figure 2. The accuracy of *BIRC5* expression in the peripheral blood for the diagnosis of endometriosis. Red dotted line indicates line of no-discrimination.

Considering the overall endometriosis group, the area under the curve (AUC) was 0.887 (95% CI = 0.809–0.965; $p < 0.001$), with a cut-off value of $2^{-\Delta Ct} > 0.00030$, 97.2% of sensitivity and specificity of 65.5%; with a positive predictive value of 68.5% (95% CI 61.0–75.2) and a negative predictive value of 92.8% (95% CI 64.2–98.9). Regarding the minimal/mild endometriosis group, the AUC presented a value of 0.925 (95% CI = 0.848–1.0; $p < 0.001$), with a cut-off value of $2^{-\Delta Ct} > 0.0018$, sensitivity of 100% and specificity of 79.3%, positive predictive value 66.7% (95% CI 49.5–80.3), and negative predictive value 100%. For the moderate/severe endometriosis group, the AUC was 0.868 (95% CI = 0.775–0.962; $p < 0.001$), with a cut-off value of $2^{-\Delta Ct} > 0.00030$, sensitivity of 95.8% and specificity of 65.5%, with a positive predictive value of 69.7% (95% CI 58.0–79.3) and a negative predictive value of 95.0% (95% CI 73.3–99.2).

4. Discussion

In the current study, the expression pattern of BIRC5 as a potential non-invasive biomarker was assessed in the peripheral blood samples taken during different phases of the menstrual cycle of women with and without endometriosis. Our results showed that BIRC5 is differently expressed in women with endometriosis compared with healthy controls, regardless of the endometriosis stage.

Some findings have highlighted the main role of inflammation in endometriosis by acting on proliferation, apoptosis, and angiogenesis. Nevertheless, the mechanisms underlying this disease are still unclear [32]. Homeostasis maintenance of tissue is mainly regulated by cell death and some studies have shown that apoptosis increases during the menstrual cycle to retain cell homeostasis, removing aged cells from the functional layer of the endometrium [33]. The rate of apoptosis is decreased in endometrial cells of women with endometriosis, and therefore, it may contribute to the pathogenesis of the disease [34–38].

In apoptosis inhibition, survivin has a key role in both intrinsic and extrinsic pathways of apoptosis [39–44]. Considering the aspects of an immune response, survivin modulates the apoptotic threshold of neutrophils and its expression increases during inflammatory reactions in these cells. Survivin has also a contribution to T-cell development, maturation, activation, and homeostasis [20,42]. Its expression increases after the activation of naive T cells in lymphoid organs, showing the importance of survivin in the initiation of immune responses. The increased level of survivin has been documented in serum and lymphocytes of patients with different autoimmune diseases [20,42,43]. Numerous studies have shown that peritoneal leukocytes and their inflammatory mediators exert local effects, creating a microenvironment that may facilitate the development and progression of endometriotic lesions. Besides, some authors have suggested that endometriosis may have, at least in part, an autoimmune component [43,44].

Zwerts et al. [45] observed that the structures of the embryo show high expression of survivin, while the absence of its expression in endothelial cells contributes to the death of the embryo. Other studies also demonstrated that the presence of survivin is essential for normal development and organogenesis. Survivin's involvement in the regulation of endothelial cell survival and its influence in maintaining vascular integrity has paramount importance in neurogenesis, angiogenesis, and cardiogenesis. The survival of undifferentiated pluripotent stem cells is highly dependent on anti-apoptotic factors, such as survivin [46,47], and overexpression of survivin in embryonic stem cells, pluripotent cells and somatic stem cells [48,49], as well as the correlation between higher BIRC5 expression and lower cell differentiation in cells derived from bone marrow [47] is probably due to the fact that bone marrow is a source of hematopoietic stem cells and mesenchymal stem cells [50,51].

All these findings corroborate different theories for the origin of endometriosis, such as the theory of endometrial stem cells [52] or the increase in transient progenitor cells in which circulating stem cells originating from bone marrow or the basal layer of the endometrium can differentiate into endometrial tissue in different anatomical locations; or the theory of genetic/epigenetic changes in which, regardless of the origin of the initial cell, genic variants or epigenetic changes associated with changes in the peritoneal environment, such as inflammatory, immunological and oxidative stress, could initiate diseases in their different forms (ovarian, peritoneal, deep, and lesions outside the pelvis) and thus explain its complexity [11,53], which may lead also to significant anatomical alterations and make the surgical approach difficult [54]. Recently, a systematic review that summarized the findings from 21 studies and 1263 women with endometriosis reported that survivin (gene and/or protein) expression is increased in endometriosis, regardless of the methodology used (real-time reverse transcription polymerase chain reaction (RT-PCR), quantitative PCR (RT-qPCR), immunohistochemistry, Western blot, or enzyme-linked immunosorbent assay (ELISA)), sample studied (endometrium or blood), the phenotype of the endometriosis (superficial, ovarian, and deep) or morphology of the endometriotic lesions (pigmented or non-pigmented) [43].

Zang et al. [28] observed that the presence of paracrine factors produced by normal endometrial stromal cells mediated the effect of progesterone on glandular endometriotic cells in vitro. The authors also found that endometriotic stromal cells have lost the ability to regulate apoptotic signaling in endometriotic gland cells that grow in ectopic sites, while these cells have not lost their ability to respond to paracrine factors produced by endometrial stromal cells. The observation of the cyclic expression of survivin in normal endometrial cells suggests that the expression of the BIRC5 gene is influenced by steroid hormones and deregulated by the increase in progesterone in the luteal phase. Progesterone is a potent antagonist of estrogen-induced endometrial proliferation and plays an important role in the pathogenesis of endometriosis [55]. The continuous use of progestogens, as well as the combined use of estrogens and progestogens in the treatment of endometriosis results in the inhibition of endometrial growth, with consequent atrophy of the lesions, in addition to being associated with anti-inflammatory action, suppression of metalloproteinases, and inhibition of angiogenesis [56]. In the present study, Spearman's correlation showed that progesterone level was correlated with BIRC5 expression (rho = 0.382, p = 0.045).

Acimovic et al. [57] studied survivin expression in 30 women with endometriosis and 10 women without the disease. The authors found a difference in the expression of survivin in peripheral blood between the groups (p = 0.025) and the results demonstrated that the accuracy of survivin as a diagnostic test for endometriosis was 70%, with a sensitivity of 66.7% and specificity of 80%. However, the study does not report the phase of the menstrual cycle during which the samples were collected. In our study, the expression of BIRC5 in the peripheral blood of women with endometriosis showed an accuracy of 88.7%, with a sensitivity of 97.2% and specificity of 65.5%. In minimum/mild endometriosis the accuracy was 92.5%, with 100% sensitivity and 79.3% specificity, whereas in moderate/severe disease the accuracy was 86.8% with 95.8% sensitivity and specificity of 65.5%. The data suggest that BIRC5 expression may be a potential minimally invasive biomarker in the diagnosis of endometriosis.

Some studies suggest that prolactin may also act as a probable prognostic biomarker to differentiate patients with endometriosis according to the stage of the disease and also as an indicator of endometriosis related-infertility since higher levels are observed in women with endometriosis when compared with infertile women without endometriosis; however, this relation is debatable [58]. Prolactin plays an important role in the immune system, participating in the inflammatory process, angiogenesis, and in the formation of thrombi and scarring [59]. In our study, we observed that women with endometriosis had higher levels of prolactin, despite being within the reference value, when compared to fertile women without the disease; in addition, we did not find a significant difference for prolactin values considering the stage of the disease (13.5 ng/mL (7.6–19.3) versus 15.2 ng/mL (10.5–20.2), respectively in minimal/mild and moderate/severe endometriosis; p = 0.410). Nonetheless, minimal/mild disease was found in only one-third of the women enrolled in this study. Indeed, 66.7% of the women in the endometriosis group were classified as advanced (III/IV) stages according to the rASRM, and this could be considered in line with the enrollment of women with endometriosis-associated infertility.

For the correct interpretation of our findings, some limitations of the present study should be taken into account. We studied infertile women with endometriosis and fertile women without the disease, and the mechanisms responsible for the association of infertility and endometriosis are still not fully elucidated. As women with endometriosis were undergoing assisted reproduction treatment and the strict inclusion and exclusion criteria of the study participants, we were unable to obtain samples from the same participant at different phases of the menstrual cycle.

5. Conclusions

In conclusion, increased expression of the BIRC5 gene in the peripheral blood of women with endometriosis may indicate their role in cell proliferation and anti-apoptotic activity in the development of the disease. The findings suggest that the expression of BIRC5 may be a potential noninvasive biomarker for the diagnosis of endometriosis.

Increased knowledge of the pathophysiologic mechanisms of endometriosis is crucial for an early and accurate diagnosis, which can reduce the costs associated with the management of the disease and help to avoid (or at least reduce) the negative impact on the physical and psychosocial health of the patients.

More studies however are needed to confirm the applicability of the proposed biomarker of endometriosis for clinical use.

Author Contributions: Conceptualization, F.L.A.F. and B.B.; Data curation, C.F., R.B., T.G.P., and C.M.T.; Formal analysis, C.F., C.M.T, and F.L.A.F.; Investigation, C.F., R.B., and F.L.A.F.; Project administration, B.B.; Validation, B.B.; Writing—original draft, C.F.; Writing—review & editing, A.S.L., R.B., T.G.P., D.M.C., C.M.T., F.L.A.F., C.P.B., and B.B. All authors have read and agreed to the published version of the manuscript.

Funding: This research received no external funding.

Acknowledgments: The authors thank CAPES for granting Carolina Filipchiuk a PhD scholarship. The authors are also grateful to the FAPESP (#2017/10045-2) for granting Rubia Beteli a scientific Initiation scholarship.

Conflicts of Interest: The authors declare no conflict of interest.

References

1. Chapron, C.; Marcellin, L.; Borghese, B.; Santulli, P. Rethinking mechanisms, diagnosis and management of endometriosis. *Nat. Rev. Endocrinol.* **2019**, *15*, 666–682. [CrossRef]
2. Zondervan, K.T.; Becker, C.M.; Koga, K.; Missmer, S.A.; Taylor, R.N.; Viganò, P. Endometriosis. *Nat. Rev. Dis. Primers* **2018**, *4*, 9. [CrossRef]
3. Kiesel, L.; Sourouni, M. Diagnosis of endometriosis in the 21st century. *Climacteric* **2019**, *22*, 296–302. [CrossRef] [PubMed]
4. Barbosa, C.P.; Souza, A.M.; Bianco, B.; Christofolini, D.; Bach, F.A.; Lima, G.R. Frequency of endometriotic lesions in peritoneum samples from asymptomatic fertile women and correlation with CA125 values. *Sao Paulo Med. J.* **2009**, *127*, 342–345. [CrossRef]
5. Bast, R.C., Jr.; Badgwell, D.; Lu, Z.; Marquez, R.; Rosen, D.; Liu, J.; Baggerly, K.A.; Atkinson, E.N.; Skates, S.; Zhang, Z.; et al. New tumor markers: CA125 and beyond. *Int. J. Gynecol. Cancer* **2005**, *15* (Suppl. 3), 274–281. [CrossRef]
6. Dunselman, G.A.; Vermeulen, N.; Becker, C.; Calhaz-Jorge, C.; D'Hooghe, T.; De Bie, B.; Heikinheimo, O.; Horne, A.W.; Kiesel, L.; Nap, A.; et al. European Society of Human Reproduction and Embryology. ESHRE guideline: Management of women with endometriosis. *Hum. Reprod.* **2014**, *29*, 400–412. [CrossRef]
7. Barra, F.; Biscaldi, E.; Scala, C.; Laganà, A.S.; Vellone, V.G.; Stabilini, C.; Ghezzi, F.; Ferrero, S. A Prospective Study Comparing Three-Dimensional Rectal Water Contrast Transvaginal Ultrasonography and Computed Tomographic Colonography in the Diagnosis of Rectosigmoid Endometriosis. *Diagnostics* **2020**, *10*, 252. [CrossRef]
8. Laganà, A.S.; Garzon, S.; Götte, M.; Viganò, P.; Franchi, M.; Ghezzi, F.; Martin, D.C. The Pathogenesis of Endometriosis: Molecular and Cell Biology Insights. *Int. J. Mol. Sci.* **2019**, *20*, 5615. [CrossRef]
9. Sofo, V.; Götte, M.; Laganà, A.S.; Salmeri, F.M.; Triolo, O.; Sturlese, E.; Retto, G.; Alfa, M.; Granese, R.; Abrão, M.S. Correlation between dioxin and endometriosis: An epigenetic route to unravel the pathogenesis of the disease. *Arch. Gynecol. Obstet.* **2015**, *292*, 973–986. [CrossRef] [PubMed]
10. Wang, Y.; Nicholes, K.; Shih, I.M. The Origin and Pathogenesis of Endometriosis. *Annu. Rev. Pathol.* **2020**, *15*, 71–95. [CrossRef]
11. Alkatout, İ.; Meinhold-Heerlein, I.; Keckstein, J.; Mettler, L. Endometriosis: A concise practical guide to current diagnosis and treatment. *J. Turk. Ger. Gynecol. Assoc.* **2018**, *19*, 173–175. [CrossRef] [PubMed]
12. Alderman, M.H.; Yoder, N.; Taylor, H.S. The Systemic Effects of Endometriosis. *Semin. Reprod. Med.* **2017**, *35*, 263–270. [CrossRef]
13. Freytag, D.; Mettler, L.; Maass, N.; Günther, V.; Alkatout, I. Uterine anomalies and endometriosis. *Minerva Med.* **2020**, *111*, 33–49. [CrossRef]
14. Melin, A.; Sparén, P.; Persson, I.; Bergqvist, A. Endometriosis and the risk of cancer with special emphasis on ovarian cancer. *Hum. Reprod.* **2006**, *21*, 1237–1242. [CrossRef]
15. Wang, C.; Liang, Z.; Liu, X.; Zhang, Q.; Li, S. The Association between Endometriosis, Tubal Ligation, Hysterectomy and Epithelial Ovarian Cancer: Meta-Analyses. *Int. J. Environ. Res. Public Health* **2016**, *13*, 1138. [CrossRef]
16. Králíčková, M.; Laganà, A.S.; Ghezzi, F.; Vetvicka, V. Endometriosis and risk of ovarian cancer: What do we know? *Arch. Gynecol. Obstet.* **2020**, *301*, 1–10. [CrossRef]

17. Moga, M.A.; Bălan, A.; Dimienescu, O.G.; Burtea, V.; Dragomir, R.M.; Anastasiu, C.V. Circulating miRNAs as Biomarkers for Endometriosis and Endometriosis-Related Ovarian Cancer-An Overview. *J. Clin. Med.* **2019**, *8*, 735. [CrossRef]
18. Karnezis, A.N.; Leung, S.; Magrill, J.; McConechy, M.K.; Yang, W.; Chow, C.; Kobel, M.; Lee, C.H.; Huntsman, D.G.; Talhouk, A.; et al. Evaluation of endometrial carcinoma prognostic immunohistochemistry markers in the context of molecular classification. *J. Pathol. Clin. Res.* **2017**, *3*, 279–293. [CrossRef]
19. Wheatley, S.P.; McNeish, I.A. Survivin: A protein with dual roles in mitosis and apoptosis. *Int. Rev. Cytol.* **2005**, *247*, 35–88. [CrossRef]
20. Zafari, P.; Rafiei, A.; Esmaeili, S.A.; Moonesi, M.; Taghadosi, M. Survivin a pivotal antiapoptotic protein in rheumatoid arthritis. *J. Cell. Physiol.* **2019**, *234*, 21575–21587. [CrossRef]
21. Marsicano, S.R.; Kuniyoshi, R.K.; Gehrke, F.S.; Alves, B.C.; Azzalis, L.A.; Fonseca, F.L. Survinin expression in patients with breast cancer during chemotherapy. *Tumour Biol.* **2015**, *36*, 3441–3445. [CrossRef] [PubMed]
22. Rivadeneira, D.B.; Caino, M.C.; Seo, J.H.; Angelin, A.; Wallace, D.C.; Languino, L.R.; Altieri, D.C. Survivin promotes oxidative phosphorylation, subcellular mitochondrial repositioning, and tumor cell invasion. *Sci. Signal.* **2015**, *8*, ra80. [CrossRef]
23. Ausserlechner, M.J.; Hagenbuchner, J. Mitochondrial survivin–an Achilles' heel in cancer chemoresistance. *Mol. Cell Oncol.* **2015**, *3*, e1076389. [CrossRef]
24. Galbo, P.M., Jr.; Ciesielski, M.J.; Figel, S.; Maguire, O.; Qiu, J.; Wiltsie, L.; Minderman, H.; Fenstermaker, R.A. Circulating CD9+/GFAP+/survivin+ exosomes in malignant glioma patients following survivin vaccination. *Oncotarget* **2017**, *8*, 114722–114735. [CrossRef]
25. Wheatley, S.P.; Altieri, D.C. Survivin at a glance. *J. Cell Sci.* **2019**, *132*, jcs223826. [CrossRef]
26. Konno, R.; Yamakawa, H.; Utsunomiya, H.; Ito, K.; Sato, S.; Yajima, A. Expression of survivin and Bcl-2 in the normal human endometrium. *Mol. Hum. Reprod.* **2000**, *6*, 529–534. [CrossRef]
27. Lehner, R.; Enomoto, T.; McGregor, J.A.; Shroyer, L.; Haugen, B.R.; Pugazhenthi, U.; Shroyer, K.R. Correlation of survivin mRNA detection with histologic diagnosis in normal endometrium and endometrial carcinoma. *Acta Obstet. Gynecol. Scand.* **2002**, *81*, 162–167. [CrossRef]
28. Zhang, H.; Li, M.; Zheng, X.; Sun, Y.; Wen, Z.; Zhao, X. Endometriotic stromal cells lose the ability to regulate cell-survival signaling in endometrial epithelial cells in vitro. *Mol. Hum. Reprod.* **2009**, *15*, 653–663. [CrossRef]
29. Takai, N.; Miyazaki, T.; Nishida, M.; Nasu, K.; Miyakawa, I. Survivin expression correlates with clinical stage, histological grade, invasive behavior and survival rate in endometrial carcinoma. *Cancer Lett.* **2002**, *184*, 105–116. [CrossRef]
30. Pallares, J.; Martínez-Guitarte, J.L.; Dolcet, X.; Llobet, D.; Rue, M.; Palacios, J.; Prat, J.; Matias-Guiu, X. Survivin expression in endometrial carcinoma: A tissue microarray study with correlation with PTEN and STAT-3. *Int. J. Gynecol. Pathol.* **2005**, *24*, 247–253. [CrossRef]
31. Canis, M.; Donnez, J.G.; Guzick, D.S.; Halme, J.K.; Rock, J.A.; Schenken, R.S.; Vernon, M.W. Revised American Society for Reproductive Medicine classification of endometriosis: 1996. *Fertil. Steril.* **1997**, *67*, 817–821. [CrossRef]
32. Burney, R.O.; Giudice, L.C. Pathogenesis and pathophysiology of endometriosis. *Fertil. Steril.* **2012**, *98*, 511–519. [CrossRef] [PubMed]
33. Vetvicka, V.; Laganà, A.S.; Salmeri, F.M.; Triolo, O.; Palmara, V.I.; Vitale, S.G.; Sofo, V.; Králíčková, M. Regulation of apoptotic pathways during endometriosis: From the molecular basis to the future perspectives. *Arch. Gynecol. Obstet.* **2016**, *294*, 897–904. [CrossRef]
34. Kokawa, K.; Shikone, T.; Nakano, R. Apoptosis in the human uterine endometrium during the menstrual cycle. *J. Clin. Endocrinol. Metab.* **1996**, *81*, 4144–4147.
35. Gebel, H.M.; Braun, D.P.; Tambur, A.; Frame, D.; Rana, N.; Dmowski, W.P. Spontaneous apoptosis of endometrial tissue is impaired in women with endometriosis. *Fertil. Steril.* **1998**, *69*, 1042–1047. [CrossRef]
36. Vaskivuo, T.E.; Stenbäck, F.; Karhumaa, P.; Risteli, J.; Dunkel, L.; Tapanainen, J.S. Apoptosis and apoptosis-related proteins in human endometrium. *Mol. Cell. Endocrinol.* **2000**, *165*, 75–83. [CrossRef]
37. Uegaki, T.; Taniguchi, F.; Nakamura, K.; Osaki, M.; Okada, F.; Yamamoto, O.; Harada, T. Inhibitor of apoptosis proteins (IAPs) may be effective therapeutic targets for treating endometriosis. *Hum. Reprod.* **2015**, *30*, 149–158. [CrossRef]
38. Vallée, A.; Lecarpentier, Y. Curcumin and Endometriosis. *Int. J. Mol. Sci.* **2020**, *21*, 2440. [CrossRef]

39. Riedl, S.J.; Shi, Y. Molecular mechanisms of caspase regulation during apoptosis. *Nat. Rev. Mol. Cell Biol.* **2004**, *5*, 897–907. [CrossRef]
40. Okada, H.; Mak, T.W. Pathways of apoptotic and non-apoptotic death in tumour cells. *Nat. Rev. Cancer* **2004**, *4*, 592–603. [CrossRef]
41. Altieri, D.C. Survivin, versatile modulation of cell division and apoptosis in cancer. *Oncogene* **2003**, *22*, 8581–8589. [CrossRef] [PubMed]
42. Altznauer, F.; Martinelli, S.; Yousefi, S.; Thürig, C.; Schmid, I.; Conway, E.M.; Schöni, M.H.; Vogt, P.; Mueller, C.; Fey, M.F.; et al. Inflammation-associated cell cycle-independent block of apoptosis by survivin in terminally differentiated neutrophils. *J. Exp. Med.* **2004**, *199*, 1343–1354. [CrossRef] [PubMed]
43. Bianco, B.; Filipchiuk, C.; Christofolini, D.M.; Barbosa, C.P.; Montagna, E. The role of survivin in the pathogenesis of endometriosis. *Minerva Med.* **2020**, *111*, 21–32. [CrossRef]
44. Matarese, G.; De Placido, G.; Nikas, Y.; Alviggi, C. Pathogenesis of endometriosis: Natural immunity dysfunction or autoimmune disease? *Trends Mol. Med.* **2003**, *9*, 223–228. [CrossRef]
45. Zwerts, F.; Lupu, F.; De Vriese, A.; Pollefeyt, S.; Moons, L.; Altura, R.A.; Jiang, Y.; Maxwell, P.H.; Hill, P.; Oh, H.; et al. Lack of endothelial cell survivin causes embryonic defects in angiogenesis, cardiogenesis, and neural tube closure. *Blood* **2007**, *109*, 4742–4752. [CrossRef]
46. Lee, M.O.; Moon, S.H.; Jeong, H.C.; Yi, J.-Y.; Lee, T.-H.; Shim, S.H.; Rhee, Y.-H.; Lee, S.-H.; Oh, S.-J.; Lee, M.-Y.; et al. Inhibition of pluripotent stem cell-derived teratoma formation by small molecules. *Proc. Natl. Acad. Sci. USA* **2013**, *110*, E3281–E3290. [CrossRef]
47. Gil-Kulik, P.; Krzyżanowski, A.; Dudzińska, E.; Karwat, J.; Chomik, P.; Świstowska, M.; Kondracka, A.; Kwaśniewska, A.; Cioch, M.; Jojczuk, M.; et al. Potential Involvement of BIRC5 in Maintaining Pluripotency and Cell Differentiation of Human Stem Cells. *Oxid. Med. Cell. Longev.* **2019**, *2019*, 8727925. [CrossRef]
48. Mull, A.N.; Klar, A.; Navara, C.S. Differential localization and high expression of SURVIVIN splice variants in human embryonic stem cells but not in differentiated cells implicate a role for SURVIVIN in pluripotency. *Stem Cell Res.* **2014**, *12*, 539–549. [CrossRef]
49. Altieri, D.C. Survivin–The inconvenient IAP. *Semin. Cell Dev. Biol* **2015**, *39*, 91–96. [CrossRef]
50. Maijenburg, M.W.; Kleijer, M.; Vermeul, K.; Mul, E.P.J.; van Alphen, F.P.J.; van der Schoot, C.E.; Voermans, C. The composition of the mesenchymal stromal cell compartment in human bone marrow changes during development and aging. *Haematologica* **2012**, *97*, 179–183. [CrossRef]
51. Reagan, M.R.; Rosen, C.J. Navigating the bone marrow niche: Translational insights and cancer-driven dysfunction. *Nat. Rev. Rheumatol.* **2016**, *12*, 154–168. [CrossRef] [PubMed]
52. Laganà, A.S.; Salmeri, F.M.; Vitale, S.G.; Triolo, O.; Götte, M. Stem Cell Trafficking During Endometriosis: May Epigenetics Play a Pivotal Role? *Reprod. Sci.* **2018**, *25*, 978–979. [CrossRef] [PubMed]
53. Koninckx, P.R.; Ussia, A.; Adamyan, L.; Wattiez, A.; Gomel, V.; Martin, D.C. Pathogenesis of endometriosis: The genetic/epigenetic theory. *Fertil. Steril.* **2019**, *111*, 327–340. [CrossRef] [PubMed]
54. Alkatout, I. Laparoscopic hysterectomy: Total or subtotal?–Functional and didactic aspects. *Minim. Invasive Ther. Allied Technol.* **2020**. [CrossRef]
55. García-Gómez, E.; Vázquez-Martínez, E.R.; Reyes-Mayoral, C.; Cruz-Orozco, O.P.; Camacho-Arroyo, I.; Cerbón, M. Regulation of Inflammation Pathways and Inflammasome by Sex Steroid Hormones in Endometriosis. *Front. Endocrinol.* **2020**, *10*, 935. [CrossRef]
56. Laschke, M.W.; Menger, M.D. Anti-angiogenic treatment strategies for the therapy of endometriosis. *Hum. Reprod. Update* **2012**, *18*, 682–702. [CrossRef]
57. Acimovic, M.; Vidakovic, S.; Milic, N.; Jeremic, K.; Markovic, M.; Milosevic-Djeric, A.; Lazovic-Radonjic, G. Survivin and VEGF as Novel Biomarkers in Diagnosis of Endometriosis. *J. Med. Biochem.* **2016**, *35*, 63–68.
58. Mirabi, P.; Alamolhoda, S.H.; Golsorkhtabaramiri, M.; Namdari, M.; Esmaeilzadeh, S. Prolactin concentration in various stages of endometriosis in infertile women. *JBRA Assist. Reprod.* **2019**, *23*, 225–229. [CrossRef]
59. Marschalek, J.; Ott, J.; Husslein, H.; Kuessel, L.; Elhenicky, M.; Mayerhofer, K.; Franz, M.B. The impact of GnRH agonists in patients with endometriosis on prolactin and sex hormone levels: A pilot study. *Eur. J. Obstet. Gynecol. Reprod. Biol.* **2015**, *195*, 156–159. [CrossRef]

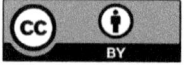

© 2020 by the authors. Licensee MDPI, Basel, Switzerland. This article is an open access article distributed under the terms and conditions of the Creative Commons Attribution (CC BY) license (http://creativecommons.org/licenses/by/4.0/).

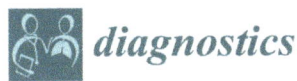

Article

Uncovering Potential Roles of Differentially Expressed Genes, Upstream Regulators, and Canonical Pathways in Endometriosis Using an In Silico Genomics Approach

Zeenat Mirza [1,2,*] and Umama A. Abdel-dayem [1,2]

1 King Fahd Medical Research Center, King Abdulaziz University, Jeddah 21589, Saudi Arabia; uabdelsalam@kau.edu.sa
2 Department of Medical Lab Technology, Faculty of Applied Medical Sciences, King Abdulaziz University, Jeddah 21589, Saudi Arabia
* Correspondence: zmirza1@kau.edu.sa

Received: 9 May 2020; Accepted: 17 June 2020; Published: 19 June 2020

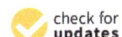

Abstract: Endometriosis is characterized by ectopic endometrial tissue implantation, mostly within the peritoneum, and affects women in their reproductive age. Studies have been done to clarify its etiology, but the precise molecular mechanisms and pathophysiology remain unclear. We downloaded genome-wide mRNA expression and clinicopathological data of endometriosis patients and controls from NCBI's Gene Expression Omnibus, after a systematic search of multiple independent studies comprising 156 endometriosis patients and 118 controls to identify causative genes, risk factors, and potential diagnostic/therapeutic biomarkers. Comprehensive gene expression meta-analysis, pathway analysis, and gene ontology analysis was done using a bioinformatics-based approach. We identified 1590 unique differentially expressed genes (129 upregulated and 1461 downregulated) mapped by IPA as biologically relevant. The top upregulated genes were *FOS*, *EGR1*, *ZFP36*, *JUNB*, *APOD*, *CST1*, *GPX3*, and *PER1*, and the top downregulated ones were *DIO2*, *CPM*, *OLFM4*, *PALLD*, *BAG5*, *TOP2A*, *PKP4*, *CDC20B*, and *SNTN*. The most perturbed canonical pathways were mitotic roles of Polo-like kinase, role of Checkpoint kinase proteins in cell cycle checkpoint control, and ATM signaling. Protein–protein interaction analysis showed a strong network association among FOS, EGR1, ZFP36, and JUNB. These findings provide a thorough understanding of the molecular mechanism of endometriosis, identified biomarkers, and represent a step towards the future development of novel diagnostic and therapeutic options.

Keywords: endometriosis; microarray; transcriptomics; biomarker; canonical pathways

1. Introduction

Endometriosis is a painful gynecological ailment marked by the presence of endometrial tissue outside the uterine cavity, commonly involving the uterus, ovaries, fallopian tubes, and pelvic tissues [1]. It is a complex and chronic estrogen-dependent disorder, wherein abnormal growth of uterine-lining (endometrium) tissue occurs outside the uterus, which can lead to serious complications like diabetes, obesity, mood disorders, dysmenorrhea, chronic pelvic pain, or even fatal endometrial cancer and cardiovascular disorders if left untreated for long. The most common site of endometriosis is the Douglas pouch (rectovaginal region) of the pelvic peritoneum [2]. Common symptoms include agonizing abdominal pain, period cramps (dysmenorrhea), heavy periods, pain with bowel movements or urination, dyspareunia, and infertility [3].

Pelvic exams and sonography are done to visualize abnormalities, and laparoscopy is required for diagnosis as well as treatment. Modes of treatment are primarily hormonal suppression and ultrasonographically guided surgical/laparoscopic management, which only provide symptomatic relief and the condition can recur with time [4]. Unfortunately, invasive surgery and the lack of a disease biomarker presently causes a mean latency of 7–11 years from symptom onset to definitive diagnosis. This substantial lag possibly has negative consequences in terms of disease progression.

An estimated 176 million women are affected by it worldwide, and studies suggest that 10% of females of reproductive age suffer from this inflammatory disorder. The prevalence of endometriosis is 11.1% among Saudi Arabian women [5]. However, the condition is often underdiagnosed and undertreated. Future higher risk for endometrial polyps [6] and rare progression to endometriosis-associated adenocarcinoma exists in endometriosis patients. They also have a lifetime predisposition to clear-cell and endometrioid types of ovarian cancer [7], which are endometriosis-derived, and which are possibly associated with retrograde menstruation [8]. The identification of a sufficiently specific and sensitive marker for the non-surgical detection of endometriosis would promise early diagnosis and prevention of detrimental effects, underscoring the need for comprehensive research. The most extensively studied potential biomarker for endometriosis is cancer antigen 125, but its use as a sole diagnostic marker is impractical due to its low sensitivity [9].

Recent innovations of high-throughput transcriptomics-based genome-wide approaches have had a major impact on medical research [10], thereby aiding in clinical classification and treatment predictions [10–12]. Understanding the genetic basis of the pathophysiology of endometriosis is important to explain the strong genetic association with heritability, estimated at around 50% [13]. Dysregulation of several genes has been implicated in the etiology of this ectopic condition.

In a menstrual cycle, endometrium undergoes transition from estrogen-dominant proliferative (follicular) phases (early-proliferative (EP), mid-proliferative (MP), and late-proliferative (LP)) to progesterone-dominant secretory (luteal) phases ((early-secretory (ES), mid-secretory (MS), and late-secretory (LS)), followed by the menstrual phase. A distinct differential transcriptional profile exists for each endometrial cycle phase [14,15]. As the uterine linings in endometriosis patients have altered transcriptomic profiles, molecular classification is needed for disease identification and staging [16]. Previous works have focused on expression profiling of different stages of the endometrial cycle in small groups. Herein, we integrated data to conduct comprehensive differential transcriptional profiling of a large cohort in order to identify differentially expressed genes, upstream regulators, and perturbed canonical pathways that could possibly be used in future to identify novel potential biomarkers and therapeutic targets for endometriosis.

Etiology

Decrease in age of menarche, fewer pregnancies, less breast feeding, and increase in maternal age at first birth all cause an overall increase in the number of ovulations and menstruations within a reproductive lifespan. These changes are associated strongly with the risk of endometriosis development and tend to be more pronounced during the decade of highest risk for endometriosis, i.e., 25–35 years of age [17]. Estrogen dependence, immune modulation, and certain environmental pollutants, mostly dioxins and polychlorinated biphenyls, perhaps contribute to the disease's pathobiology [18]. Immunological or hormonal dysfunction make some women predisposed to endometriosis. Higher macrophage activation and humoral immune responsiveness with reduced cell-mediated immunity, with weakened T-cell and NK-cell responses, are seen in women suffering from endometriosis. Humoral autoantibodies against endometrial and ovarian tissue have been detected in endometriosis patient sera [19].

The pathogenesis of endometriosis has been speculated to result from aberrant angiogenesis that occurs in the eutopic endometrium with retrograde menstruation—"Sampson's hypothesis" [2]. Factors that increase the rate of retrograde menstruation, such as congenital outflow tract obstructions, might also predispose to endometriosis. Detailed understanding on the basis of gene expression studies is lacking, and findings are often inconsistent or even contradictory.

2. Materials and Methods

2.1. Data Retrieval and Sample Description

Our approach was the integration of publicly available gene expression data generated by different microarray platforms. We first retrieved whole-transcript array datasets (.CEL files) along with provided clinical details of endometriosis patients dated up to 30 March 2020 from the Gene Expression Omnibus (GEO, NCBI) databank, a public domain hosting high-throughput genomic data. The present study included following expression data series with GEO accession numbers GSE7846, GSE7305, GSE6364, GSE4888, GSE51981, GSE31683, and GSE25628 and their sample information to compare the transcriptomic status of affected and control patients (Table 1). The GSE51981 dataset has a total of 148 endometrial samples from patients with ages ranging from 20–50 years. It includes samples from women in different menstrual cycle phases, including endometriosis with severe pelvic pain/infertility ($n = 77$) and normal without endometriosis ($n = 71$). Normal women with uterine fibroids, adenomyosis, or pelvic organ prolapse were further grouped as normal with uterine/pelvic pathology ($n = 37$), and others as normal without uterine pathology ($n = 34$). The GSE7846 dataset includes five arrays for human endometrial endothelial cells (HEECs) derived from eutopic endometria of patients with endometriosis, and five from patients without endometriosis (controls). GSE7305 includes expression profiles of 10 each of normal and diseased cases.

2.2. Gene Expression Analysis

To generate expression profiles of endometriosis samples, .CEL files were imported to Partek Genomics Suite, version 7.0 (Partek Inc., St. Louis, MO, USA) followed by log-transformation and normalization of the robust background-adjusted array dataset. Principal component analysis (PCA) was done on high-dimensional data to assess quality and overall variance in gene expression of individuals among sample groups. Analysis of variance (ANOVA) was employed to create a list of differentially expressed genes (DEGs) with a cut-off p-value of ≤ 0.05 and fold change of ± 2. Hierarchical clustering was done to reveal the pattern of most differentially expressed (up- and downregulated) genes across samples.

2.3. Gene Ontology, Pathway, and Upstream Regulators Analysis

The identified statistically significant DEGs with corresponding probe sets ID, p-value, fold-change values, and other relevant data were uploaded into the Ingenuity Pathways Analysis (IPA, QIAGEN's Ingenuity Systems, Redwood City, CA, USA) software for molecular network and canonical pathway analysis to define interaction amongst the differentially regulated genes using functional algorithms. The Benjamini–Hochberg method was used to adjust p-values for canonical pathways, and p-values below 0.01 and Altman z-scores of ± 2 were considered significant. Positive and negative values of z-score represent activation and inhibition of dysregulated canonical pathways. Gene ontology study was done to functionally categorize endometriosis-significant genes. All endometriosis-associated DEGs were imported to figuratively represent all identified connections and potential relationships among them, in order to identify significant pathways leading to endometriosis initiation and progression.

2.4. Protein–Protein Interaction Analysis

To check the interactions at the protein level, the STRING v11.0 database (http://string-db.org) was used to search for possible physical and functional associations among proteins encoded by the top DEGs (including both up- and downregulated) for a better understanding of disease pathobiology [20]. This prediction gives a visual idea about the possible interconnections between the proteins involved in a specific disease network.

3. Results

Differentially Expressed Genes from Meta-Analysis

Integration of the seven GEO data series included in present study comprised a total of 156 endometriosis patients and 118 controls. Data were merged before analysis as all had used the same GPL570 platform, except GSE25628 which used the GPL571 platform (Table 1).

Table 1. Gene expression Omnibus (GEO) data series, platform, and sample description of endometrium-based expression studies (total 156 endometriosis patients + 118 normal cases).

GEO Data Series	Total No. of Cases (Diseased + Normal)	Platform	Sample Description
GSE 7846	10 (5 + 5)	GPL570	Endometriosis ($n = 5$), Normal ($n = 5$)
GSE 7305	20 (10 + 10)	GPL570	Endometriosis ($n = 10$), Normal ($n = 10$)
GSE 6364	37 (21 + 16)	GPL570	Proliferative ($n = 6$), Proliferative normal ($n = 5$); Early-secretory ($n = 6$), Early-secretory normal ($n = 3$); Mid-secretory ($n = 9$), Mid-secretory normal ($n = 8$)
GSE 4888	27 (21 + 6)	GPL570	Proliferative ($n = 4$), Early-secretory ($n = 3$), Mid-secretory ($n = 8$), Late-secretory ($n = 6$), Ambiguous histology ($n = 6$)
GSE 51981	148 (77 + 71)	GPL570	Severe endometriosis ($n = 48$), Mild endometriosis ($n = 29$), Normal without pelvic/uterine pathology ($n = 34$), Normal with pelvic/uterine pathology ($n = 37$)
GSE 31683	10 (6 + 4)	GPL570	*KLF9* silenced ($n = 2$), *PGR* silenced ($n = 2$), Both *KLF9* and *PGR* silenced ($n = 2$), Normal ($n = 4$)
GSE 25628	22 (16 + 6)	GPL571	Eutopic ($n = 9$), Ectopic ($n = 7$), Normal ($n = 6$)

Principal component analysis showed the grouping of the samples in three-dimensional space as per their whole-genome expression patterns, where each circle represents an individual (Figure 1). Comparing endometriosis with normal non-endometriosis tissue without any pelvic/uterine pathology resulted in the detection of 1590 differentially expressed genes (129 upregulated and 1461 downregulated). The top upregulated genes, including *FOS, EGR1, ZFP36, JUNB, APOD, CST1, GPX3,* and *PER1*, are shown in Table 2 and the top downregulated genes, including *DIO2, CPM, OLFM4, PALLD, BAG5, TOP2A, PKP4, CDC20B,* and *SNTN*, are shown in Table 3. Hierarchical clustering of DEGs showed a clear difference in expression pattern of genes between endometriosis cases and controls (Figure 2). Disease and functional annotation of DEGs broadly predicted endometrial adenocarcinoma. However, DEGs like *FOS, EGR1, ZFP36, JUNB, GPX3, PAEP, DUSP1, MT1M, COL6A1, NR4A1, TGFB1, CITED2, IL2RG, ACKR1, JUN, PTGER3, COL6A2, PGR, PLK2, PLA2G4A, FBN1, MPPED2, EZR, MMP11, GALNT4, PTEN, PIK3CA, CREB1, ERBIN, DNMT3A, REL, SDC2, ZNF25, ITGA6, GUCY1A2, PDGFD, OVGP1, ITGB1, APOBEC3B, OLFM1, NRIP1, MEF2A, CNTN1, BUB1B, MEST, KIF20A, RRM1, ANK3,* and *CCNA2* showed significant association with endometriosis (p-value = 0.0006).

Ingenuity pathway analysis for the DEGs of endometriosis revealed altered canonical pathways that were either activated or inhibited (Figure 3, Table 4). Mitotic roles of polo-like kinase (z-score −2.71), aldosterone signaling in epithelial cells (z-score −3.464), and role of CHK proteins in cell cycle checkpoint control (z-score −0.632) were found to be inhibited while ATM signaling (z-score + 1.698) and SUMOylation pathways (z-score + 2.668) were activated (Figure 4, Figure 5). IPA predicted the activation status of upstream regulators among identified DEGs of endometriosis. REL (transcription factor, z-score −4.13, Pval 0.0002), CTNNB1 (transcription factor, z-score −3.2, Pval 0.01), PGR (ligand-dependent nuclear receptor, z-score −2.2, Pval 0.0005), and VCAN (proteoglycan, z-score −2.6, Pval 0.02) were the top inhibited upstream regulators (Table 5). We also used a biological database, STRING, to predict functional associations and interaction between the proteins encoded by the identified significant DEGs (top up- and downregulated ones), and the results are shown in

Figure 6. The network indicated a strong interplay of various proteins and their specific involvement in endometriosis.

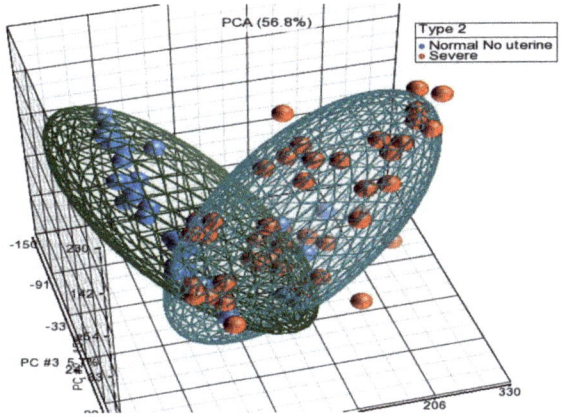

Figure 1. PCA showing two clear distinct clusters for severe endometriosis cases and normal healthy controls without uterine pathology.

Table 2. Top overexpressed/upregulated differentially expressed genes in endometriosis.

Gene Symbol	Gene Name	p-Value	Fold-Change
FOS	FBJ murine osteosarcoma viral oncogene homolog	3.02×10^{-13}	9.94558
EGR1	early growth response 1	7.67×10^{-17}	7.95823
FOSB	FBJ murine osteosarcoma viral oncogene homolog B	1.87×10^{-10}	7.14284
ZFP36	ZFP36 ring finger protein	5.23×10^{-14}	4.01565
JUNB	jun B proto-oncogene	8.28×10^{-15}	4.01404
APOD	apolipoprotein D	1.21×10^{-7}	3.7376
CST1	cystatin SN	2.52×10^{-5}	3.42216
GPX3	glutathione peroxidase 3	0.0057	3.34348
PER1	period circadian clock 1	6.14×10^{-13}	3.23599
CTSW	cathepsin W	8.08×10^{-7}	3.22223
SOCS3	suppressor of cytokine signaling 3	4.99×10^{-5}	3.11348
CFD	complement factor D (adipsin)	0.000993	2.99141
HSPB6	heat shock protein, alpha-crystallin-related, B6	9.31×10^{-8}	2.98362
LEFTY1	left-right determination factor 1	0.004712	2.89285
PAEP	progestagen-associated endometrial protein	0.029113	2.88223
DUSP1	dual specificity phosphatase 1	1.48×10^{-7}	2.88219
GNLY	Granulysin	1.52×10^{-5}	2.83639
EPHX1	epoxide hydrolase 1, microsomal (xenobiotic)	6.69×10^{-10}	2.78618
MT1M	metallothionein 1M	0.011648	2.76574
CLEC3B///EXOSC7	C-type lectin domain family 3, member B///exosome component 7	7.13×10^{-5}	2.74002
GNLY	Granulysin	1.61×10^{-5}	2.73433
TPSAB1///TPSB2	tryptase alpha/beta 1///tryptase beta 2 (gene/pseudogene)	1.20×10^{-6}	2.73381
IER2	immediate early response 2	4.65×10^{-14}	2.67138
PTPRO	protein tyrosine phosphatase, receptor type, O	2.70×10^{-14}	2.66719
ELN	Elastin	2.26×10^{-7}	2.6637
IER3	immediate early response 3	5.70×10^{-5}	2.61981
SOX13	SRY box 13	4.59×10^{-9}	2.60666
SOD3	superoxide dismutase 3, extracellular	2.00×10^{-9}	2.60457
SLC30A2	solute carrier family 30 (zinc transporter), member 2	0.002566	2.59508
AQP3	aquaporin 3 (Gill blood group)	0.000604	2.58706
HSPB6	heat shock protein, alpha-crystallin-related, B6	2.81×10^{-6}	2.57421
CD37	CD37 molecule	3.56×10^{-8}	2.48625
IRX3	iroquois homeobox 3	0.00585	2.48441
CREB3L1	cAMP responsive element binding protein 3-like 1	1.53×10^{-7}	2.48023

Table 3. The top downregulated differentially expressed genes in meta-analysis of endometriosis.

Gene Symbol	Gene Title	p-Value	Fold-Change
DIO2	deiodinase, iodothyronine, type II	6.84×10^{-12}	−5.38638
CPM	carboxypeptidase M	1.52×10^{-7}	−5.20763
OLFM4	olfactomedin 4	1.22×10^{-6}	−4.77761
PALLD	palladin, cytoskeletal associated protein	1.20×10^{-13}	−4.47775
BAG5	BCL2-associated athanogene 5	1.62×10^{-8}	−4.38993
TOP2A	topoisomerase (DNA) II alpha	4.50×10^{-8}	−4.22713
PKP4	plakophilin 4	5.35×10^{-19}	−3.97475
CDC20B	cell division cycle 20B	1.36×10^{-6}	−3.96043
SNTN	sentan, cilia apical structure protein	5.43×10^{-12}	−3.95899
SET	SET nuclear proto-oncogene	5.39×10^{-11}	−3.90488
CRISPLD1	cysteine-rich secretory protein LCCL domain containing 1	5.12×10^{-7}	−3.85982
NPAS3	neuronal PAS domain protein 3	1.57×10^{-6}	−3.83298
CADM1	cell adhesion molecule 1	4.63×10^{-15}	−3.78248
SMC3	structural maintenance of chromosomes 3	2.59×10^{-16}	−3.7407
SFRP4	secreted frizzled-related protein 4	0.000481	−3.72407
ANK2	ankyrin 2, neuronal	2.00×10^{-7}	−3.71876
ANLN	anillin actin binding protein	4.54×10^{-8}	−3.70838
WIF1	WNT inhibitory factor 1	1.73×10^{-6}	−3.65345
MMP26	matrix metallopeptidase 26	0.002107	−3.63998
PCSK5	proprotein convertase subtilisin/kexin type 5	7.33×10^{-8}	−3.63558
OXR1	oxidation resistance 1	1.62×10^{-13}	−3.61905
CTNNB1	catenin (cadherin-associated protein), beta 1	6.39×10^{-12}	−3.55057
PCSK5	proprotein convertase subtilisin/kexin type 5	1.69×10^{-8}	−3.53439
EIF5B	eukaryotic translation initiation factor 5B	1.60×10^{-8}	−3.52153
HSP90B1	heat shock protein 90kDa beta (Grp94), member 1	2.11×10^{-9}	−3.49988
PCYOX1	prenylcysteine oxidase 1	3.06×10^{-11}	−3.47374
MIB1	mindbomb E3 ubiquitin protein ligase 1	1.96×10^{-9}	−3.46544
OSBPL1A	oxysterol binding protein-like 1A	2.08×10^{-14}	−3.46429
CBX3	chromobox homolog 3	2.18×10^{-12}	−3.45307
TCAF1	TRPM8 channel-associated factor 1	1.87×10^{-13}	−3.42665
KMO	kynurenine 3-monooxygenase (kynurenine 3-hydroxylase)	2.06×10^{-5}	−3.42531
CTSZ	cathepsin Z	3.75×10^{-13}	−3.40201
KMO	kynurenine 3-monooxygenase (kynurenine 3-hydroxylase)	2.13×10^{-5}	−3.38857
PCSK5	proprotein convertase subtilisin/kexin type 5	5.06×10^{-8}	−3.38299
YWHAB	tyrosine 3-monooxygenase/tryptophan 5-monooxygenase activation protein, beta	2.64×10^{-13}	−3.35541
NMT2	N-myristoyltransferase 2	5.60×10^{-12}	-3.34186
CADM1	cell adhesion molecule 1	3.18×10^{-9}	−3.3281
CEP57	centrosomal protein 57kDa	3.21×10^{-15}	−3.28628

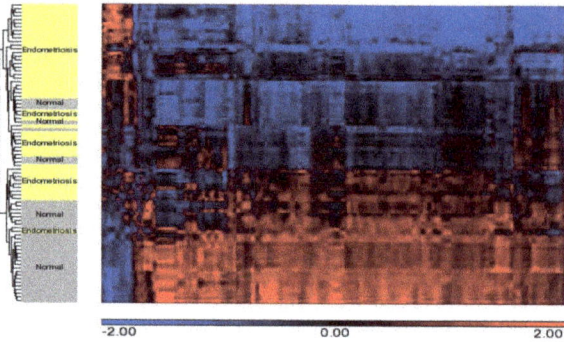

Figure 2. Hierarchical clustering showing distribution of DEGs and cases. Downregulated and upregulated genes are shown in blue and red, respectively, showing a distinct pattern with a majority of genes found to be downregulated in endometriosis.

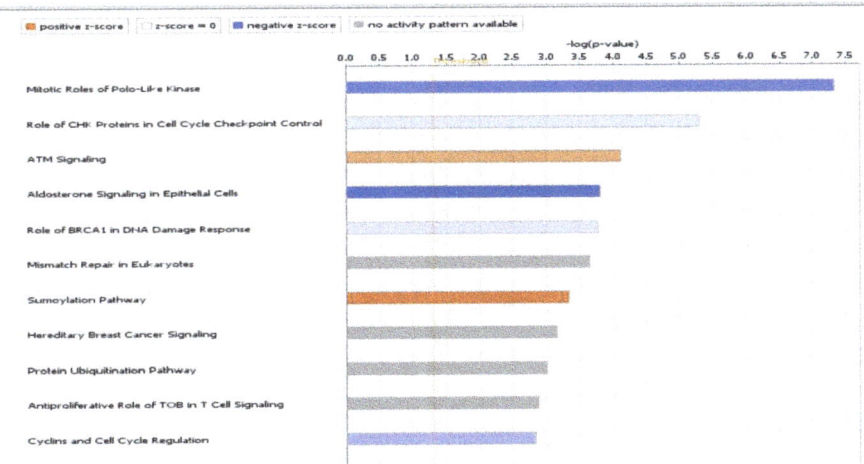

Figure 3. Significant pathways identified by IPA. The top 11 altered canonical pathways predicted from DEGs of endometriosis. Negative and positive z-scores, colored in shades of blue and red, represent inhibition and activation of pathways, respectively.

Table 4. Significant canonical pathways based on DEGs of endometriosis. Positive and negative z- scores indicate overall activation and inhibition status of pathways, respectively.

Ingenuity Canonical Pathways	−log (p-Value)	Ratio	Predicted z-Score	Molecules
Mitotic Roles of Polo-Like Kinase	7.34	0.333	−2.714 (Inhibited)	ANAPC4, CCNB1, CCNB2, CDC23, CDC27, CDK1, FBXO5, HSP90AA1, HSP90AB1, HSP90B1, KIF11, KIF23, PLK2, PPM1L, PPP2R2C, PPP2R5C, PPP2R5E, PRC1, RAD21, SMC3, TGFB1
ATM Signaling	4.11	0.219	1.698 (Activated)	ATF1, CBX1, CBX3, CBX5, CCNB1, CCNB2, CDK1, CHEK1, CREB1, FANCD2, JUN, PPM1L, PPP2R2C, PPP2R5C, PPP2R5E, RAD17, RAD50, SMC2, SMC3, TLK1, ZNF420
Aldosterone Signaling in Epithelial Cells	3.8	0.183	−3.464 (Inhibited)	DNAJA1, DNAJB14, DNAJC10, DNAJC27, DNAJC3, DNAJC9, DUSP1, HSP90AA1, HSP90B1, HSPA4, HSPA9, HSPB6, HSPD1, HSPH1, ITPR2, PDIA3, PDPK1, PIK3C2A, PIK3CA, PIK3R3, PIP5K1B, PLCB1, PRKCI, PRKD3, SACS, SCNN1G
Role of CHK Proteins in Cell Cycle Checkpoint Control	5.3	0.298	−0.632	ATMIN, CDK1, CHEK1, E2F7, E2F8, PCNA, PPM1L, PPP2R2C, PPP2R5C, PPP2R5E, RAD17, RAD50, RFC3, RFC4, RFC5, RPA1, TLK1
SUMOylation Pathway	3.34	0.198	2.668 (Activated)	DNMT3A, EP300, FOS, HDAC2, JUN, MYB, PCNA, PIAS1, RFC3, RFC4, RFC5, RHOB, RHOBTB1, RHOQ, RHOT1, RND3, RPA1, SERBP1, SMAD4, UBA2
Role of BRCA1 in DNA Damage Response	3.77	0.225	−0.707	ABRAXAS1, ATF1, BRCC3, BRD7, BRIP1, CHEK1, E2F7, E2F8, FANCD2, FANCL, MSH2, MSH6, RAD50, RFC3, RFC4, RFC5, RPA1, SMARCC1
Cyclins and Cell Cycle Regulation	2.83	0.2	−1.604	CCNA1, CCNA2, CCNB1, CCNB2, CCNE2, CDK1, CDK6, E2F7, E2F8, HDAC2, PPM1L, PPP2R2C, PPP2R5C, PPP2R5E, SKP2, TGFB1
PI3K/AKT Signaling	2.7	0.171	−1.091	CTNNB1, EIF4E, HSP90AA1, HSP90AB1, HSP90B1, INPP5F, ITGB1, JAK1, PDPK1, PIK3CA, PIK3R3, PPM1L, PPP2R2C, PPP2R5C, PPP2R5E, PTEN, RASD1, RHEB, RPS6KB1, SFN, SYNJ2, YWHAB

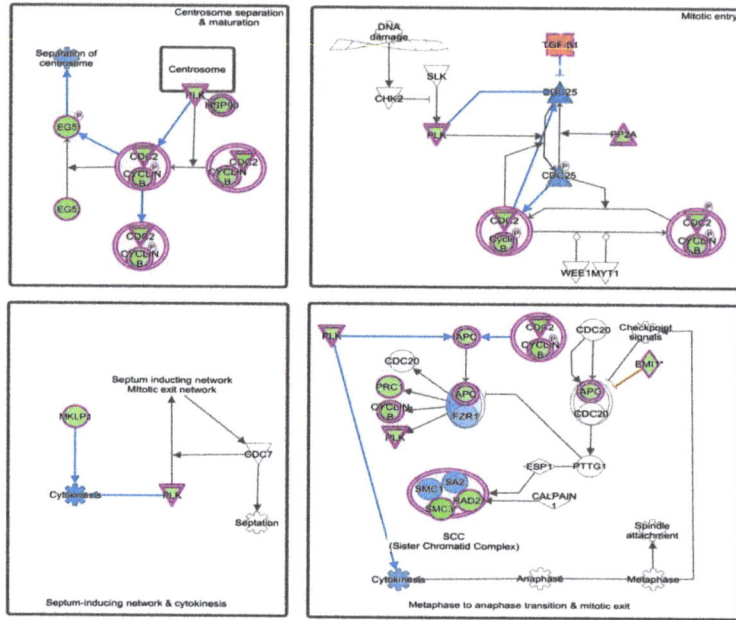

Figure 4. Significant inhibition of mitotic polo-like kinase pathway predicted by IPA. Pathway genes were overlaid to the DEGs; upregulated (*TGFB1*, *CDC25*, *FZR1*) genes are shown in red/pink, while downregulated genes (*PRC1*, *PLK*, *Cyclin B1*, *SMC3*) are shown in green.

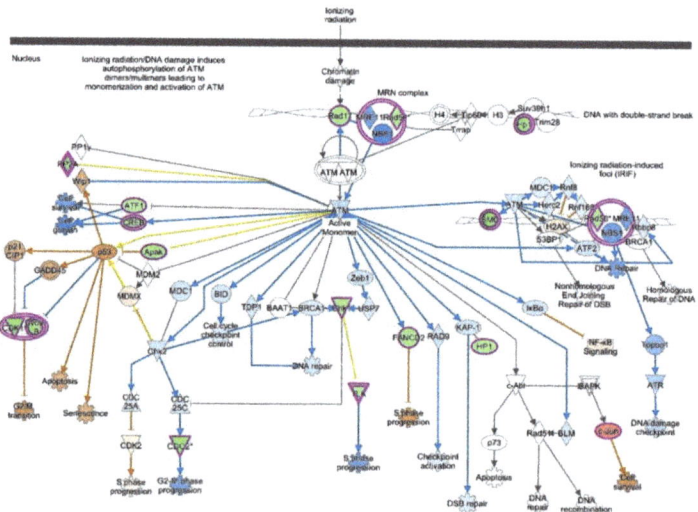

Figure 5. Activation of ATM signaling predicted by IPA-based pathway analysis. Pathway genes were overlaid to the DEGs, with upregulated ones shown in shades of red and downregulated ones shown in green.

Table 5. Most significant upstream regulators and target molecules in endometriosis dataset.

Upstream Regulator	Molecule Type	Predicted Activation z-score	p-Value of Overlap	Target Molecules in Dataset
REL	transcription regulator	−4.137 (Inhibited)	0.00021	AGA, AGPS, ANLN, APP, ARFGAP3, ATXN1, BCL3, CAMK2D, CCNY, CDC6
CTNNB1	transcription regulator	−3.208 (Inhibited)	0.0104	AKAP13, ALDH1A1, APOD, APP, ARFGAP3, ARMH4, AURKA, CADM1, CALM1, CCL3
PGR	ligand-dependent nuclear receptor	−2.237 (Inhibited)	0.00051	ABCG2, ACOX1, AHCYL1, AK3, AKAP13, ATP1B1, ATXN1, BUB1, CA12, CCNB1
VCAN	Proteoglycan	−2.625 (Inhibited)	0.024	COMP, CPE, ELN, IFI44L, IFIT1, ITGB1, MYH10, PCSK5, PENK, PLA2G2A
ACTL6A	Other	−2.236 (Inhibited)	0.093	CCNA2, CCNB1, CCNB2, CCNE2, SFN
DUSP1	phosphatase	−2.155 (Inhibited)	1	CMPK2, DUSP1, IER3, IFIT1, IFIT3, JUN, PTEN, ZFP36
HELLS	Enzyme	−2 (Inhibited)	0.0024	CCNA2, CCNB1, CDC6, HSPD1, PCNA, SLC44A1
RASSF8	Other	−2 (Inhibited)	0.0016	ENPP5, MRPL30, NEDD9, POSTN
TCF4	transcription regulator	−1.912	0.040	CCNA2, CCNB2, CDK1, CEP55, E2F8, FOS, HMGB2, HMMR, HSP90B1, IFI16
IGF2R	transmembrane receptor	−2 (Inhibited)	0.0080	ENPP5, MRPL30, NEDD9, POSTN
TGFB1	growth factor	−1.276	0.00087	ABCG2, ACKR1, ADAM12, ALDH5A1, APP, ARHGAP19, ASPM, ATG12, ATXN1, BCL3
HSF2	transcription regulator	−1.408	0.026	CCT2, HSBP1, HSPA4, HSPH1, JUN, PSMA5, TCP1
EDN3	other	0.816	0.0024	CDH2, CTNNB1, EGR1, FOS, ITGB1, LAMA1
FOS	transcription regulator	0.917	0.0020	ACOX1, ADAM12, AGPS, ANK3, AQP3, ATP2C1, CADM1, CALU, CAMK2D, CAT
RTN4	other	1.51	0.0041	APP, CFL1, IMPACT, JUN, JUND, LAP3, MAP2, RHOB, RTN4, YWHAB
ZFP36	transcription regulator	1.873	0.00015	CCNE2, CDC6, CENPA, CLCN3, CLMP, CTSS, E2F8, FOS, IER3, JUN
EPHB1	kinase	1.98	0.0052	EGR1, FOS, JUN, JUNB

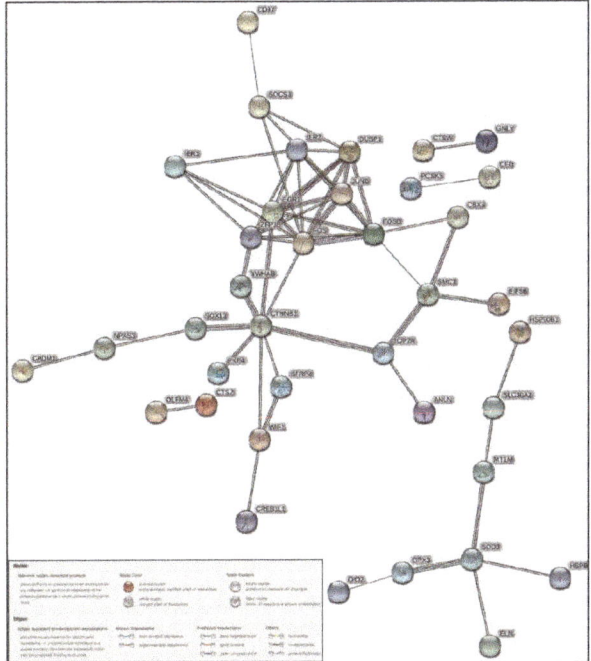

Figure 6. STRING-based protein–protein interaction (PPI) network of selected differentially expressed genes, showing predicted interconnectivities.

4. Discussion

Endometriosis, a growth/deposition of endometrial tissue at extra-uterine sites, affects around 10% of reproductive women. In addition to abnormal reproductive physiological problems, cases are increasing drastically due to adverse consequences of treatment with oral contraceptives, GnRH agonists, synthetic progestins, and aromatase inhibitors (letrozole) to prevent the menstrual cycle and/or pregnancy [1,21]. Understanding the molecular etiology of origin and progression of endometriosis is necessary to explore therapeutic options and provide better treatment. We therefore conducted transcriptomic meta-analysis to identify endometriosis-associated significant DEGs and essential pathological pathways.

Combining multiple studies has always been challenging, as different studies use varied protocols, platforms, and analysis methods. We used raw data (.CEL) files to integrate multiple data series to get a bigger cohort and analyzed the data. We identified transcriptomic signatures of endometriosis and evaluated the roles of specific genes, upstream regulators, and dysregulated pathways. Our results provide some insight into the molecular mechanisms underlying endometriosis pathogenesis. Pathogenic genes and pathways may serve as novel targets for diagnostic and prognostic biomarkers and potential therapies for endometriosis. In the present study, we had a long list of genes and pathways, but have restricted our discussion to the most prominent genes and pathways.

4.1. Molecular Etiology of Endometriosis

Retrograde or "reverse" menstruation has been suggested as an initial cause of endometriosis, where menstrual blood is thrown back into pelvic cavity outside the uterus, instead of flowing out of the cervix. This endometrial tissue growth out of the uterus is the result of an estrogen-dependent hormonal local imbalance. Higher prevalence has been also seen in women with immune disorders (like rheumatoid arthritis, multiple sclerosis, systemic lupus erythematosus, and hypo- or hyperthyroidism) [17]. Recently, a small-molecule agonist G-1 (Tespria) against the G-protein-coupled estrogen receptor also showed reduction in endometrial growth [22].

Unusual transformation of certain abdominal wall cells into endometrial cells has been reported in some women [23] and, interestingly, it is believed that during embryonic development, the same cells are responsible for the growth of female reproductive organs. Researchers also think that pelvic inflammation, damage, or infection of cells that line the pelvis like a prior caesarean surgery can also trigger endometriosis [23–25]. The exact pathogenesis still remains uncertain. We therefore conducted a transcriptomics study in order to understand the genetic factors that allow cells to grow as endometrial tissue outside the uterus.

In our results, we found high expression of early and immediate early-response genes such as FBJ murine osteosarcoma viral oncogene homolog or *Fos proto-Oncogene (FOS)*, *FosB Proto-Oncogene (FOSB)*, *Early Growth Response 1 (EGR1)*, *ZFP36 Ring Finger Protein (ZFP36)*, *Immediate Early Response 2 (IER2)*, *Immediate Early Response 3 (IER3)*, *Jun B Proto-Oncogene (JUNB)*, and *Transcription Factor SOX-13 (SOX 13)*. The majority of these are DNA-binding proteins that act as transcriptional factors. Some others, like *Dual specificity protein phosphatase 1 (DUSP1)* and *Receptor-type tyrosine-protein phosphatase O (PTPRO)*, possess phosphatase activity.

c-Fos is the transcription factor of the Fos family, including *FosB*, *Fra-1*, and *Fra-2* [26]. It is an immediate early-response gene involved in cell proliferation and differentiation of normal tissue after extracellular stress stimuli. Its deregulation has been linked to oncogenic transformation and tumor progression. *FOS* plays a significant role in endometrial cells' proliferation and its overexpression is associated with a poor prognosis of endometrial carcinoma [27]. Fos and Jun family proteins form a heterodimer complex of AP-1 transcription factor, shown to be involved in endometrial carcinogenesis [28]. Upstream regulator analysis revealed genes such as *REL*, *CTNNB1*, *PGR*, and *VCAN* by analyzing linkage to DEGs that were experimentally shown to affect gene expression [29]. All upstream regulators were inhibited.

REL: *REL* (*V-Rel Avian Reticuloendotheliosis Viral Oncogene Homolog*) encodes for the proto-oncogene c-Rel protein, a transcription factor of the NF-κB family that regulates genes involved in B- and T-cell differentiation, immune response, survival, apoptosis, proliferation, and oncogenic processes, including endometrial carcinogenesis [30,31].

CTNNB1: *CTNNB1* (*Catenin β1*) codes for a protein that regulates and coordinates cell–cell adhesion, embryonic development, epithelial–mesenchymal transition, and gene transcription. It is an integral part of the canonical Wnt pathway. Aberrant Wnt/β-catenin signaling pathway function is allied with loose cytoskeleton organization and cell-to-cell contacts of epithelial cells, along with a high motility of mesenchymal cells to promote invasiveness and fibrosis. This might lead to multiple cancers, including endometrial cancer [32–36]. Targeting the Wnt/β-catenin signaling was shown to avert fibrogenesis in a xenograft endometriosis mice model [35].

VCAN: *VCAN* (*Versican*) codes for four extracellular matrix isoforms like large chondroitin sulfate proteoglycan in different tissues and organs that regulate cell adhesion, proliferation, migration, and survival [2]. Higher expression of *VCAN* has been reported in angiogenesis, tumor growth, cancer relapse, and inflammatory lung disorders [37–39]. Significantly high expression of *VCAN* was also reported in the mid-secretory phase of endometrial epithelial cells after combination estrogen/progesterone treatment. The V1 isoform of *VCAN* was recently reported to the facilitate development of endometrial receptivity and human embryo implantation [40]. Higher expression of *VCAN* is connected with pathogenesis of peritoneal endometriosis and seems to be an indicator of poor prognosis endometrial cancer [2,41].

Alteration in expression of *HOXB4* [42], apelin peptide [43], interleukin 18 [44], estrogen and progesterone receptors [45], integrin β3 and osteopontin (*OPN*) [46], microRNA-29c, and FKBP4 [47] have been reported. Varied expression levels of metastasis-inducing proteins (*S100P*, *S100A4*, *OPN*, and anterior gradient homologue 2 (*AGR2*)) have been shown to enhance pathogenesis by increasing endometrial cell invasiveness and establishing endometriotic ectopic deposits after retrograde menstruation [48].

Aromatase activates estrogen biosynthesis locally from androgens, thereby sequentially stimulating a positive feedback cycle of prostaglandin E2 production by upregulating cyclooxygenase-2 (*COX-2*). Because of lack of aromatase (estrogen synthase) in the normal endometrium, androgens cannot be converted into estrogen [49]. In contrast, numerous studies have described aberrantly high expression of aromatase in eutopic and ectopic endometrium [17]. Increased *COX-2* expression in the stromal cells and aberrant aromatase overexpression in eutopic endometrium have both been indicated as potential therapeutic biomarkers, and therefore, their specific inhibitors are being increasingly employed for therapeutic management [50]. A probable connection of Krüppel-like Factor 9 (*KLF9*) dysregulation has been suggested in both pregnancy failure and endometrial pathogenesis [51]. The progesterone resistance and subsequent infertility seen in endometriosis seems to have an association with *KLF9*, a progesterone-receptor-interacting protein, as mice null for Klf9 are sub-fertile. It is implicated that deficiency of *KLF9* contributes to progesterone resistance of eutopic endometrium in patients [52] and exhibits simultaneous abrogation of Hedgehog-, Notch-, and steroid-receptor-regulated networks [53].

Based on serum proteomic differential expression, a possible biomarker panel comprising zinc-alpha-2-glycoprotein, albumin, and complement C3 has been proposed for effective and non-invasive diagnosis of endometriosis [54]. Importantly, the three markers were independent from the endometriosis stage and cycle phase. Brain Derived Neurotrophic Factor (*BDNF*) has been identified as a potential peripheral early diagnostic marker, as its mean plasma concentrations were twice as high in endometriosis cases in contrast to asymptomatic or healthy controls [9]. Based on this, a nano-chip-based electrochemical detection technique was developed. The only limitation to this is its non-specificity, as the variations in *BDNF* expression have been reported in numerous unconnected pathologies [55].

4.2. Canonical Pathways Involved in Endometriosis

Molecular pathway analysis revealed a couple of significantly altered canonical pathways for DEGs of endometriosis. Herein, we discuss the role of key pathways like Mitotic roles of polo-like kinase, Role of CHK proteins in cell cycle checkpoint control, Aldosterone signaling in epithelial cells, and ATM Signaling in endometriosis progression.

Mitotic Roles of Polo-Like Kinase Pathway: The Polo-like kinase (Plks) is a member of the serine/threonine protein kinase (*PLK1-5*) family that regulates the mitotic checkpoint during M phase of cell division. Plks can act either as oncogene or tumor suppressor, and has been found to be overexpressed in different cancer types including endometrial [56] and ovarian [57] cancers. Because of its direct association with increased cellular proliferation and poor prognosis, it is considered a bona fide cancer biomarker [58,59]. Direct association of Plks expression with serum estrogen (ovarian hormone) levels and abnormal regulation of ectopic endometrial cell proliferation strongly suggest its role in the pathogenesis of endometriosis [60]. Plks inhibitors such as volasertib and rigosertib are in advanced stage of clinical trials and might be used for endometriosis treatment [61].

Role of CHK Proteins in Cell Cycle Checkpoint Control Pathway: Activation of cell cycle checkpoint kinases including Chk1 and Chk2 are an instant response to repair any type of DNA damage [62]. In response to DNA damage, this signaling pathway temporarily delays cell cycle progression, allowing time for DNA repair, or triggers programmed cell death. Activated ATM kinase phosphorylates Chk2 which phosphorylates *CDC25C* to block the progression from G2 to M phase. Chk2 also phosphorylates p53, attenuating p53 binding to *MDM2* and activating p21/WAF1 to arrest the G1 phase of the cell cycle. *Rad3*-dependent activation of Chk1 phosphorylates *CDC25A* and *CDC2* to inhibit their activity to block G2–M transition. Overall, CHK protein signaling depends on the type of stress and extent of DNA damage and is involved in endometrial cancer [63].

Cisplatin exerts an anticancer effect by activating DNA-damage-response genes Chk1/2, which generates both survival (repair) and apoptotic signals that lead to cell death. Cisplatin-resistant cells have dominant repair signaling that allows cells to survive. Chk1/2 inhibitor AZD7762 has been shown to overcome cisplatin resistance in endometriosis-associated ovarian cancer by reducing repair signaling [64].

ATM Signaling Pathway: Ataxia telangiectasia mutated (*ATM*) gene codes for serine/threonine protein kinase and participates in cell division and DNA repair. DNA damage induces autophosphorylation of ATM which activates DNA repair enzymes by phosphorylating Chk1/2 to fix the broken strands [65]. Efficient cross-talk between ATR-Chk1 and ATM-Chk2 leads to repair of damaged DNA strands which helps to maintain the cell's genomic stability and integrity [66]. The ATM signaling pathway, because of its central role in cell division and DNA repair, has been a focus of cancer research, especially endometrial cancer, for exploring novel molecular therapies targeting ATM pathways [67].

Aldosterone Signaling in Epithelial Cells Pathway: Aldosterone is a mineralocorticoid steroid hormone produced by the adrenal cortex. Aldosterone signaling primarily controls blood pressure and inflammation by regulating its target genes (*FKBP5*, *IGF1*, *KRAS*, *PKCε*, *NCOA1*, *NCOR1*, *NEDD4L*, *SGK*, and *MR/NR3C2* as per RGD, https://rgd.mcw.edu [68] and IPA). Recent studies have shown the possible involvement of aldosterone in multiple gynecological problems and inflammatory disorders [69]. There is a well-established association of endometriosis with intraperitoneal inflammation diseases like atherosclerosis and hypertension, and also with autoimmune diseases like diabetes, hypothyroidism, and cancer [9]. A metabolomics-based study revealed high aldosterone levels in endometriosis patients with infertility [70].

4.3. Future Directions

The strength of present work lies in the inclusion of multiple endometriosis-related expression datasets in order to understand endometriosis at the molecular level. However, the absence of a validation study was its limitation. In future, we plan to conduct RT-PCR-based validation studies for differentially expressed genes on endometriosis samples collected from the Jeddah region. Further cell cultures and animal models could be used to assess the effect of activated/suppressed genes on molecular pathways and disease phenotypes for potential clinical translation. Virtual screening of potential lead compounds against identified therapeutic biomarkers for rational drug design will be done. This could facilitate imminent tailor-made personalized therapies.

5. Conclusions

Endometriosis is an estrogen-dependent, progesterone-resistant, inflammatory multifactorial gynecological disorder. Identification of distinct molecular signatures and potential therapeutic molecules corresponding to endometriosis is needed for better diagnosis. The present microarray-based genomics and molecular pathway analysis method helped to establish a better understanding of endometriosis at the molecular level, as multiple expression datasets were integrated to determine differentially expressed genes and identify canonical molecular pathways related to endometriosis in a broad way. The study identified alterations of gene expression and molecular signaling, including aldosterone signaling, that result in the hormonal imbalances and pathogenesis of endometriosis. An anti-inflammatory diet and increased levels of antioxidants and phytonutrients can be recommended to patients to reverse inflammation and oxidative damage, while also supporting healthy hormone balance.

Author Contributions: Z.M. and U.A.A.-D. Study design, U.A.A.-D. Acquisition of data, Z.M. Analysis and interpretation of data, Z.M. Manuscript writing, U.A.A.-D. Critical review of manuscript. All authors have read and agreed to the published version of the manuscript.

Funding: This Project was funded by the Deanship of Scientific Research (DSR), King Abdulaziz University, Jeddah, under grant no. 31217 (Code: G: 500-141-1439). The authors, therefore, acknowledge and thanks DSR for its technical and financial support.

Conflicts of Interest: The authors declare no conflict of interest.

References

1. Cho, Y.J.; Lee, S.H.; Park, J.W.; Han, M.; Park, M.J.; Han, S.J. Dysfunctional signaling underlying endometriosis: Current state of knowledge. *J. Mol. Endocrinol.* **2018**, *60*, R97–R113. [CrossRef]
2. Tani, H.; Sato, Y.; Ueda, M.; Miyazaki, Y.; Suginami, K.; Horie, A.; Konishi, I.; Shinomura, T. Role of Versican in the Pathogenesis of Peritoneal Endometriosis. *J. Clin. Endocrinol. Metab.* **2016**, *101*, 4349–4356. [CrossRef] [PubMed]
3. Alimi, Y.; Iwanaga, J.; Loukas, M.; Tubbs, R.S. The Clinical Anatomy of Endometriosis: A Review. *Cureus* **2018**, *10*, e3361. [CrossRef] [PubMed]
4. Yeung, P., Jr. The laparoscopic management of endometriosis in patients with pelvic pain. *Obstet. Gynecol. Clin. N. Am.* **2014**, *41*, 371–383. [CrossRef] [PubMed]
5. Rouzi, A.A.; Sahly, N.; Kafy, S.; Sawan, D.; Abduljabbar, H. Prevalence of endometriosis at a university hospital in Jeddah, Saudi Arabia. *Clin. Exp. Obstet. Gynecol.* **2015**, *42*, 785–786.
6. Zheng, Q.M.; Mao, H.I.; Zhao, Y.J.; Zhao, J.; Wei, X.; Liu, P.S. Risk of endometrial polyps in women with endometriosis: A meta-analysis. *Reprod. Biol. Endocrinol.* **2015**, *13*, 103. [CrossRef]
7. Kim, H.S.; Kim, T.H.; Chung, H.H.; Song, Y.S. Risk and prognosis of ovarian cancer in women with endometriosis: A meta-analysis. *Br. J. Cancer* **2014**, *110*, 1878–1890. [CrossRef]
8. Vaughan, S.; Coward, J.I.; Bast, R.C.; Berchuck, A.; Berek, J.S.; Brenton, J.D.; Coukos, G.; Crum, C.C.; Drapkin, R.; Etemadmoghadam, D.; et al. Rethinking ovarian cancer: Recommendations for improving outcomes. *Nat. Rev. Cancer* **2011**, *11*, 719–725. [CrossRef]
9. Hughes, C.; Foster, W.; Agarwal, S. The impact of endometriosis across the lifespan of women: Foreseeable research and therapeutic prospects. *Biomed. Res. Int.* **2015**, *2015*, 158490. [CrossRef]
10. Sorlie, T.; Tibshirani, R.; Parker, J.; Hastie, T.; Marron, J.S.; Nobel, A.; Deng, S.; Johnsen, H.; Pesich, R.; Geisler, S.; et al. Repeated observation of breast tumor subtypes in independent gene expression data sets. *Proc. Natl. Acad. Sci. USA* **2003**, *100*, 8418–8423. [CrossRef]

11. Hedenfalk, I.; Duggan, D.; Chen, Y.; Radmacher, M.; Bittner, M.; Simon, R.; Meltzer, P.; Gusterson, B.; Esteller, M.; Kallioniemi, O.P.; et al. Gene-expression profiles in hereditary breast cancer. *N. Engl. J. Med.* **2001**, *344*, 539–548. [CrossRef] [PubMed]
12. Chang, J.C.; Wooten, E.C.; Tsimelzon, A.; Hilsenbeck, S.G.; Gutierrez, M.C.; Elledge, R.; Mohsin, S.; Osborne, C.K.; Chamness, G.C.; Allred, D.C.; et al. Gene expression profiling for the prediction of therapeutic response to docetaxel in patients with breast cancer. *Lancet* **2003**, *362*, 362–369. [CrossRef]
13. Borghese, B.; Zondervan, K.T.; Abrao, M.S.; Chapron, C.; Vaiman, D. Recent insights on the genetics and epigenetics of endometriosis. *Clin. Genet.* **2017**, *91*, 254–264. [CrossRef] [PubMed]
14. Ponnampalam, A.P.; Weston, G.C.; Trajstman, A.C.; Susil, B.; Rogers, P.A.W. Molecular classification of human endometrial cycle stages by transcriptional profiling. *Mol. Hum. Reprod.* **2004**, *10*, 879–893. [CrossRef] [PubMed]
15. Sherwin, R.; Catalano, R.; Sharkey, A. Large-scale gene expression studies of the endometrium: What have we learnt? *Reproduction* **2006**, *132*, 1–10. [CrossRef]
16. Miller, L.M.; Johnson, N.P. EPHect—The Endometriosis Phenome (and Biobanking) Harmonisation Project—May be very helpful for clinicians and the women they are treating. *F1000Res* **2017**, *6*, 14. [CrossRef]
17. Parazzini, F.; Vercellini, P.; Pelucchi, C. Endometriosis: Epidemiology, and Etiological Factors. In *Endometriosis*; Linda, C.G., Johannes, L.H.E., David, L.H., Eds.; Wiley-Blackwell: Oxford, UK, 2012; pp. 19–26. [CrossRef]
18. Porpora, M.G.; Resta, S.; Fuggetta, E.; Storelli, P.; Megiorni, F.; Manganaro, L.; De Felip, E. Role of environmental organochlorinated pollutants in the development of endometriosis. *Clin. Exp. Obstet. Gynecol.* **2013**, *40*, 565–567.
19. Mathur, S.; Peress, M.R.; Williamson, H.O.; Youmans, C.D.; Maney, S.A.; Garvin, A.J.; Rust, P.F.; Fudenberg, H.H. Autoimmunity to endometrium and ovary in endometriosis. *Clin. Exp. Immunol.* **1982**, *50*, 259–266. [CrossRef]
20. Szklarczyk, D.; Gable, A.L.; Lyon, D.; Junge, A.; Wyder, S.; Huerta-Cepas, J.; Simonovic, M.; Doncheva, N.T.; Morris, J.H.; Bork, P.; et al. STRING v11: Protein-protein association networks with increased coverage, supporting functional discovery in genome-wide experimental datasets. *Nucleic Acids Res.* **2019**, *47*, D607–D613. [CrossRef]
21. Attar, E.; Bulun, S.E. Aromatase inhibitors: The next generation of therapeutics for endometriosis? *Fertil. Steril.* **2006**, *85*, 1307–1318. [CrossRef]
22. Sharma, G.; Hu, C.; Staquicini, D.I.; Brigman, J.L.; Liu, M.; Mauvais-Jarvis, F.; Pasqualini, R.; Arap, W.; Arterburn, J.B.; Hathaway, H.J. Preclinical efficacy of the GPER-selective agonist G-1 in mouse models of obesity and diabetes. *Sci. Transl. Med.* **2020**, *12*. [CrossRef] [PubMed]
23. Marques, C.; Silva, T.S.; Dias, M.F. Clear cell carcinoma arising from abdominal wall endometriosis - Brief report and review of the literature. *Gynecol. Oncol. Rep.* **2017**, *20*, 78–80. [CrossRef] [PubMed]
24. Yıldırım, D.; Tatar, C.; Doğan, O.; Hut, A.; Dönmez, T.; Akıncı, M.; Toptaş, M.; Bayık, R.N. Post-cesarean scar endometriosis. *Turk. J. Obstet. Gynecol.* **2018**, *15*, 33–38. [CrossRef] [PubMed]
25. Sosa-Durán, E.E.; Aboharp-Hasan, Z.; Mendoza-Morales, R.C.; García-Rodríguez, F.M.; Jiménez-Villanueva, X.; Peñavera-Hernández, J.R. Clear cell adenocarcinoma arising from abdominal wall endometriosis. *Cirugía Cir.* **2016**, *84*, 245–249. [CrossRef] [PubMed]
26. Milde-Langosch, K. The Fos family of transcription factors and their role in tumourigenesis. *Eur. J. Cancer* **2005**, *41*, 2449–2461. [CrossRef] [PubMed]
27. Nemos, C.; Delage-Mourroux, R.; Jouvenot, M.; Adami, P. Onset of direct 17-beta estradiol effects on proliferation and c-fos expression during oncogenesis of endometrial glandular epithelial cells. *Exp. Cell Res.* **2004**, *296*, 109–122. [CrossRef]
28. Mahner, S.; Baasch, C.; Schwarz, J.; Hein, S.; Wölber, L.; Jänicke, F.; Milde-Langosch, K. C-Fos expression is a molecular predictor of progression and survival in epithelial ovarian carcinoma. *Br. J. Cancer* **2008**, *99*, 1269–1275. [CrossRef]
29. Krämer, A.; Green, J.; Pollard, J., Jr.; Tugendreich, S. Causal analysis approaches in ingenuity pathway analysis. *Bioinformatics* **2014**, *30*, 523–530. [CrossRef]
30. Gilmore, T.D.; Gerondakis, S. The c-Rel Transcription Factor in Development and Disease. *Genes Cancer* **2011**, *2*, 695–711. [CrossRef]
31. Pallares, J.; Martínez-Guitarte, J.L.; Dolcet, X.; Llobet, D.; Rue, M.; Palacios, J.; Prat, J.; Matias-Guiu, X. Abnormalities in the NF-κB family and related proteins in endometrial carcinoma. *J. Pathol.* **2004**, *204*, 569–577. [CrossRef]

32. Lecarpentier, Y.; Schussler, O.; Hébert, J.-L.; Vallée, A. Multiple Targets of the Canonical WNT/β-Catenin Signaling in Cancers. *Front. Oncol.* **2019**, *9*. [CrossRef] [PubMed]
33. Morin, P.J. beta-catenin signaling and cancer. *Bioessays News Rev. Mol. Cell. Dev. Biol.* **1999**, *21*, 1021–1030. [CrossRef]
34. Chen, Y.; Song, W. Wnt/catenin β1/microRNA 183 predicts recurrence and prognosis of patients with colorectal cancer. *Oncol Lett.* **2018**, *15*, 4451–4456. [CrossRef] [PubMed]
35. Matsuzaki, S.; Darcha, C. Involvement of the Wnt/beta-Catenin Signaling Pathway in the Cellular and Molecular Mechanisms of Fibrosis in Endometriosis. *PLoS ONE* **2013**, *8*, e76808. [CrossRef] [PubMed]
36. Yang, Y.-M.; Yang, W.-X. Epithelial-to-mesenchymal transition in the development of endometriosis. *Oncotarget* **2017**, *8*, 41679–41689. [CrossRef]
37. Kischel, P.; Waltregny, D.; Dumont, B.; Turtoi, A.; Greffe, Y.; Kirsch, S.; De Pauw, E.; Castronovo, V. Versican overexpression in human breast cancer lesions: Known and new isoforms for stromal tumor targeting. *Int. J. Cancer* **2010**, *126*, 640–650. [CrossRef]
38. Du, W.W.; Yang, W.; Yee, A.J. Roles of versican in cancer biology—Tumorigenesis, progression and metastasis. *Histol. Histopathol.* **2013**, *28*, 701–713. [CrossRef]
39. Andersson-Sjöland, A.; Hallgren, O.; Rolandsson, S.; Weitoft, M.; Tykesson, E.; Larsson-Callerfelt, A.K.; Rydell-Törmänen, K.; Bjermer, L.; Malmström, A.; Karlsson, J.C.; et al. Versican in inflammation and tissue remodeling: The impact on lung disorders. *Glycobiology* **2015**, *25*, 243–251. [CrossRef]
40. Miyazaki, Y.; Horie, A.; Tani, H.; Ueda, M.; Okunomiya, A.; Suginami, K.; Kondoh, E.; Baba, T.; Konishi, I.; Shinomura, T.; et al. Versican V1 in human endometrial epithelial cells promotes BeWo spheroid adhesion in vitro. *Reproduction* **2019**, *157*, 53. [CrossRef]
41. Kodama, J.; Kusumoto, T.; Seki, N.; Matsuo, T.; Ojima, Y.; Nakamura, K.; Hongo, A.; Hiramatsu, Y. Prognostic significance of stromal versican expression in human endometrial cancer. *Ann. Oncol.* **2007**, *18*, 269–274. [CrossRef]
42. AlKusayer, G.M.; Pon, J.R.; Peng, B.; Klausen, C.; Lisonkova, S.; Kinloch, M.; Yong, P.; Muhammad, E.M.S.; Leung, P.C.K.; Bedaiwy, M.A. HOXB4 Immunoreactivity in Endometrial Tissues From Women With or Without Endometriosis. *Reprod. Sci.* **2017**. [CrossRef]
43. Ozkan, Z.S.; Cilgin, H.; Simsek, M.; Cobanoglu, B.; Ilhan, N. Investigation of apelin expression in endometriosis. *J. Reprod. Infertil.* **2013**, *14*, 50–55.
44. Luo, Q.; Ning, W.; Wu, Y.; Zhu, X.; Jin, F.; Sheng, J.; Huang, H. Altered expression of interleukin-18 in the ectopic and eutopic endometrium of women with endometriosis. *J. Reprod. Immunol.* **2006**, *72*, 108–117. [CrossRef] [PubMed]
45. Jones, R.K.; Bulmer, J.N.; Searle, R.F. Immunohistochemical characterization of proliferation, oestrogen receptor and progesterone receptor expression in endometriosis: Comparison of eutopic and ectopic endometrium with normal cycling endometrium. *Hum. Reprod.* **1995**, *10*, 3272–3279. [CrossRef] [PubMed]
46. Xiao, Y.; Yang, X.L.; Sun, X.; Peng, C.; Li, X.; Wang, M.; Zhou, Y.F. [Expression of integrin beta3 and osteopontin in endometrium of patients with adenomyosis]. *Zhonghua Fu Chan Ke Za Zhi* **2009**, *44*, 354–358. [PubMed]
47. Joshi, N.R.; Miyadahira, E.H.; Afshar, Y.; Jeong, J.W.; Young, S.L.; Lessey, B.A.; Serafini, P.C.; Fazleabas, A.T. Progesterone Resistance in Endometriosis Is Modulated by the Altered Expression of MicroRNA-29c and FKBP4. *J. Clin. Endocrinol. Metab.* **2017**, *102*, 141–149. [CrossRef] [PubMed]
48. Hapangama, D.K.; Raju, R.S.; Valentijn, A.J.; Barraclough, D.; Hart, A.; Turner, M.A.; Platt-Higgins, A.; Barraclough, R.; Rudland, P.S. Aberrant expression of metastasis-inducing proteins in ectopic and matched eutopic endometrium of women with endometriosis: Implications for the pathogenesis of endometriosis. *Hum. Reprod.* **2012**, *27*, 394–407. [CrossRef] [PubMed]
49. Bulun, S.E.; Yang, S.; Fang, Z.; Gurates, B.; Tamura, M.; Zhou, J.; Sebastian, S. Role of aromatase in endometrial disease. *J. Steroid Biochem. Mol. Biol.* **2001**, *79*, 19–25. [CrossRef]
50. Ebert, A.D.; Bartley, J.; David, M. Aromatase inhibitors and cyclooxygenase-2 (COX-2) inhibitors in endometriosis: New questions—Old answers? *Eur. J. Obstet. Gynecol. Reprod. Biol.* **2005**, *122*, 144–150. [CrossRef]
51. Simmen, F.A.; Su, Y.; Xiao, R.; Zeng, Z.; Simmen, R.C.M. The Krüppel-like factor 9 (KLF9) network in HEC-1-A endometrial carcinoma cells suggests the carcinogenic potential of dys-regulated KLF9 expression. *Reprod. Biol. Endocrinol.* **2008**, *6*, 41. [CrossRef]

52. Pabona, J.M.; Simmen, F.A.; Nikiforov, M.A.; Zhuang, D.; Shankar, K.; Velarde, M.C.; Zelenko, Z.; Giudice, L.C.; Simmen, R.C. Kruppel-like factor 9 and progesterone receptor coregulation of decidualizing endometrial stromal cells: Implications for the pathogenesis of endometriosis. *J. Clin. Endocrinol. Metab.* **2012**, *97*, E376–E392. [CrossRef] [PubMed]
53. Heard, M.E.; Simmons, C.D.; Simmen, F.A.; Simmen, R.C. Kruppel-like factor 9 deficiency in uterine endometrial cells promotes ectopic lesion establishment associated with activated notch and hedgehog signaling in a mouse model of endometriosis. *Endocrinology* **2014**, *155*, 1532–1546. [CrossRef] [PubMed]
54. Signorile, P.G.; Baldi, A. Looking for an effective and non-invasive diagnostic test for endometriosis: Where are we? *Ann. Transl. Med.* **2018**, *17*, S106. [CrossRef] [PubMed]
55. Bockaj, M.; Fung, B.; Tsoulis, M.; Foster, W.G.; Soleymani, L. Method for Electrochemical Detection of Brain Derived Neurotrophic Factor (BDNF) in Plasma. *Anal. Chem.* **2018**, *90*, 8561–8566. [CrossRef] [PubMed]
56. Takai, N.; Miyazaki, T.; Fujisawa, K.; Nasu, K.; Hamanaka, R.; Miyakawa, I. Polo-like kinase (PLK) expression in endometrial carcinoma. *Cancer Lett.* **2001**, *169*, 41–49. [CrossRef]
57. Takai, N.; Miyazaki, T.; Fujisawa, K.; Nasu, K.; Hamanaka, R.; Miyakawa, I. Expression of polo-like kinase in ovarian cancer is associated with histological grade and clinical stage. *Cancer Lett.* **2001**, *164*, 41–49. [CrossRef]
58. de Cárcer, G. The Mitotic Cancer Target Polo-Like Kinase 1: Oncogene or Tumor Suppressor? *Genes* **2019**, *10*, 208. [CrossRef]
59. Fu, Z.; Wen, D. The Emerging Role of Polo-Like Kinase 1 in Epithelial-Mesenchymal Transition and Tumor Metastasis. *Cancers (Basel)* **2017**, *9*, 131. [CrossRef]
60. Tang, L.; Wang, T.-T.; Wu, Y.-T.; Zhou, C.-Y.; Huang, H.-F. High expression levels of cyclin B1 and Polo-like kinase 1 in ectopic endometrial cells associated with abnormal cell cycle regulation of endometriosis. *Fertil. Steril.* **2009**, *91*, 979–987. [CrossRef]
61. Gutteridge, R.E.A.; Ndiaye, M.A.; Liu, X.; Ahmad, N. Plk1 Inhibitors in Cancer Therapy: From Laboratory to Clinics. *Mol. Cancer Ther.* **2016**, *15*, 1427–1435. [CrossRef]
62. Zhou, B.-B.S.; Elledge, S.J. The DNA damage response: Putting checkpoints in perspective. *Nature* **2000**, *408*, 433–439. [CrossRef] [PubMed]
63. Vassileva, V.; Millar, A.; Briollais, L.; Chapman, W.; Bapat, B. Genes involved in DNA repair are mutational targets in endometrial cancers with microsatellite instability. *Cancer Res.* **2002**, *62*, 4095–4099. [PubMed]
64. Itamochi, H.; Nishimura, M.; Oumi, N.; Kato, M.; Oishi, T.; Shimada, M.; Sato, S.; Naniwa, J.; Sato, S.; Kudoh, A.; et al. Checkpoint Kinase Inhibitor AZD7762 Overcomes Cisplatin Resistance in Clear Cell Carcinoma of the Ovary. *Int. J. Gynecol. Cancer* **2014**, *24*, 61–69. [CrossRef] [PubMed]
65. Daniel, J.A.; Pellegrini, M.; Lee, J.-H.; Paull, T.T.; Feigenbaum, L.; Nussenzweig, A. Multiple autophosphorylation sites are dispensable for murine ATM activation in vivo. *J. Cell. Biol.* **2008**, *183*, 777–783. [CrossRef] [PubMed]
66. Smith, J.; Mun Tho, L.; Xu, N.; A. Gillespie, D. Chapter 3—The ATM–Chk2 and ATR–Chk1 Pathways in DNA Damage Signaling and Cancer. In *Advances in Cancer Research*; Vande Woude, G.F., Klein, G., Eds.; Academic Press: Cambridge, MA, USA, 2010; Volume 108, pp. 73–112.
67. Takeuchi, M.; Tanikawa, M.; Nagasaka, K.; Oda, K.; Kawata, Y.; Oki, S.; Agapiti, C.; Sone, K.; Miyagawa, Y.; Hiraike, H.; et al. Anti-Tumor Effect of Inhibition of DNA Damage Response Proteins, ATM and ATR, in Endometrial Cancer Cells. *Cancers (Basel)* **2019**, *11*, 1913. [CrossRef] [PubMed]
68. Smith, J.R.; Hayman, G.T.; Wang, S.J.; Laulederkind, S.J.F.; Hoffman, M.J.; Kaldunski, M.L.; Tutaj, M.; Thota, J.; Nalabolu, H.S.; Ellanki, S.L.R.; et al. The Year of the Rat: The Rat Genome Database at 20: A multi-species knowledgebase and analysis platform. *Nucleic Acids Res.* **2020**, *48*, D731–D742. [CrossRef]
69. Sabbadin, C.; Andrisani, A.; Ambrosini, G.; Bordin, L.; Donà, G.; Manso, J.; Ceccato, F.; Scaroni, C.; Armanini, D. Aldosterone in Gynecology and Its Involvement on the Risk of Hypertension in Pregnancy. *Front. Endocrinol.* **2019**, *10*, 575. [CrossRef]
70. Letsiou, S.; Peterse, D.P.; Fassbender, A.; Hendriks, M.M.; van den Broek, N.J.; Berger, R.; Dorien, F.O.; Vanhie, A.; Vodolazkaia, A.; Van Langendonckt, A.; et al. Endometriosis is associated with aberrant metabolite profiles in plasma. *Fertil. Steril.* **2017**, *107*, 699–706.e696. [CrossRef]

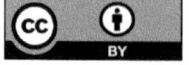

© 2020 by the authors. Licensee MDPI, Basel, Switzerland. This article is an open access article distributed under the terms and conditions of the Creative Commons Attribution (CC BY) license (http://creativecommons.org/licenses/by/4.0/).

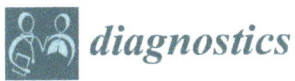

Brief Report

Microbiome Profile of Deep Endometriosis Patients: Comparison of Vaginal Fluid, Endometrium and Lesion

Camila Hernandes [1,*], **Paola Silveira** [2], **Aline Fernanda Rodrigues Sereia** [2], **Ana Paula Christoff** [2], **Helen Mendes** [1], **Luiz Felipe Valter de Oliveira** [2] **and Sergio Podgaec** [1]

1. Hospital Israelita Albert Einstein, Av. Albert Einstein 627, Morumbi, São Paulo 05651-901, Brazil; helen2002@me.com (H.M.); sergiopodgaec@me.com (S.P.)
2. BiomeHub, Av. Luiz Boiteux Piazza, 1302, Canasvieiras, Florianópolis 88056-000, Brazil; paola@biome-hub.com (P.S.); aline@biome-hub.com (A.F.R.S.); anachff@biome-hub.com (A.P.C.); felipe@biome-hub.com (L.F.V.d.O.)
* Correspondence: camila.hernandes@einstein.br; Tel.: +55-11-215-1031

Received: 1 February 2020; Accepted: 14 March 2020; Published: 17 March 2020

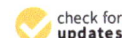

Abstract: This work aimed to identify and compare the bacterial patterns present in endometriotic lesions, eutopic endometrium and vaginal fluid from endometriosis patients with those found in the vaginal fluid and eutopic endometrium of control patients. Vaginal fluid, eutopic endometrium and endometriotic lesions were collected. DNA was extracted and the samples were analyzed to identify microbiome by high-throughput DNA sequencing of the 16S rRNA marker gene. Amplicon sequencing from vaginal fluid, eutopic endometrium and endometriotic lesion resulted in similar profiles of microorganisms, composed most abundantly by the genus *Lactobacillus*, *Gardnerella*, *Streptococcus* and *Prevotella*. No significant differences were found in the diversity analysis of microbiome profiles between control and endometriotic patients; however deep endometriotic lesions seems to present different bacterial composition, less predominant of *Lactobacillus* and with more abundant *Alishewanella*, *Enterococcus* and *Pseudomonas*.

Keywords: vaginal fluid; microbiome; next generation sequencing (NGS); pathogenesis; endometriosis; 16S rRNA

1. Introduction

Endometriosis is a gynecological disorder affecting 10% to 15% of women in reproductive age; up to 70% of the patients have pelvic pain and 48% have fertility problems [1,2]. The disease is characterized by the presence of stromal and/or endometrial glandular epithelium outside the uterus and is classified in three different types: superficial, ovarian and deep endometriosis [3–5]. Endometriosis was first described in the seventeenth century and, despite all research efforts in the last 30 years, its pathogenesis is still unclear [6].

Nowadays the most accepted hypothesis is that the foci of endometriosis originate from retrograde menstruation [7]. According to this theory, initially proposed by Sampson, the retrograde tubal flow seeds menstrual endometrial tissue in the peritoneal cavity and other organs, to which it adheres. However, as around 90% of women have retrograde menstruation, and just only 10% develop the disease, several authors have been proposed that other factors like anatomical, genetic, endocrine, environmental and inflammatory may influence this tissue implantation [8–16].

One of the most described are the inflammatory factors. Several studies have already demonstrated, for example, that the peritoneal fluid of women with endometriosis has high levels of pro-inflammatory cytokines and growth factors, such as TNF-α, IL-1 and IL-6. In previous studies carried out by our research group, we described the role of inflammatory factors presented in peritoneal fluid in the immune balance of patients with endometriosis, showing an increase in the cytokines IL-2, IL-6 and TGF-β, an increase in amyloid protein A (SAA), as well as an increase in CD4(+)CD25(high)Foxp3(+) cells, and a decrease in ICOS+Treg (T regulatory cells) and CD45RO+Treg cells in patients with the disease [10,11,14].

This inflammatory process found in patients with endometriosis has been described because it is possibly related to the presence of microorganisms. Several authors have shown, for example, an increase in the cytokine IL-1β in patients with endometriosis and they correlate this increase with the activation of inflammasomes by stimulating microorganisms, and also correlate the participation of this event in the pathogenesis of the disease [17–19].

Several other studies shown the presence of microorganisms in menstrual blood, peritoneal fluid and vagino-uterine tract [20–24], but no work so far has described the presence of microorganisms in endometriotic lesions, and their correlation with microorganisms found in vaginal secretion and eutopic endometrium.

In this context, the present project aimed to investigate, by using high-throughput DNA sequencing, the microbiome profile present in vaginal fluid, endometrium and deep endometriotic lesions of women with endometriosis in comparison to microbiome profile found in vaginal fluid and endometrium of women without the disease. As there is a lack of understanding of the relationship between them, identifying endometriosis-associated microbiome profiles could help the understanding of pathogenesis and eventually could lead to the development of a noninvasive test for endometriosis.

2. Materials and Methods

2.1. Sample Collection

This case-control study was conducted as a pilot investigation at Hospital Israelita Albert Einstein (HIAE), São Paulo, Brazil, and the protocol was approved on December, 2017 by the Research Ethics Committee of Hospital Israelita Albert Einstein (project number 80280317.5.0000.0071); all patients provided written informed consent.

Twenty-one patients were included in the study according to the inclusion and exclusion criteria outlined below. Patients were assigned to the endometriosis group after lesion(s) identification by laparoscopic surgery, and further confirmation by histopathology analysis. Just women showing deep endometriosis were included. The control group consisted of women who underwent laparoscopic surgery for benign gynecologic diseases or elective tubal ligation in which peritoneal cavity inspection confirmed absence of endometriosis.

Women aged 18–50 years presenting eumenorrheic cycles were included in the study, whether or not under hormonal treatment. Women previously diagnosed with autoimmune, inflammatory and/or neoplastic disease, and who had used antibiotics/antimycotics in the 30 days prior to samples' collection were excluded.

Eutopic endometrium and endometriotic lesion tissue samples were collected by curettage and laparoscopic surgery, respectively. All samples were collected at the operative room to minimize contamination and every care was taken to prevent the swab from touching other tissues adjacent to the target site, not having contact with blood, or any other instrument. Tissue samples were immediately frozen in liquid nitrogen and maintained at −80 °C. Vaginal fluid was sampled with sterile nylon flock swabs (Copan, Murrieta, CA, USA), also did not touched other sites and it was maintained in a microbiome transport solution (BiomeHub, Florianópolis, SC, Brazil) which allows a stable transport at ambient temperatures.

2.2. DNA Extraction and 16S rRNA Amplicon Sequencing

DNA from tissue samples was extracted using the DNeasy Power Soil Kit (QIAGEN). Processing of all samples was carried out under sterile conditions. The tissue fragments were initially minced and submitted to mechanical disruption; the DNA extraction followed the manufacturer's protocol. Vaginal fluid samples in transport solution were extracted using the QIAamp DNA Blood Mini Kit (QIAGEN) according to the manufacturer instructions. Negative control samples were included for the extraction procedures, to evaluate kit reagent DNA background and possible process contaminations.

Preparation of an amplicon sequencing library for bacteria was performed using the V3-V4 16S rRNA gene primers 341F (CCTACGGGRSGCAGCAG) [25] and 806R (GGACTACHV GGGTWTCTAAT) [26], under the following conditions: the first PCR primers contained the Illumina sequences based on TruSeq structure adapter (Illumina, San Diego, CA, USA), allowing the second PCR with indexing sequences. The PCR reactions were always carried out in triplicates using Platinum Taq (Invitrogen, Waltham, MA, USA) with the conditions: 95 °C for 5 min, 25 cycles of 95 °C for 45 s, 55 °C for 30 s and 72 °C for 45s and a final extension of 72 °C for 2 min for PCR 1. In PCR 2 the conditions were 95 °C for 5 min, 10 cycles of 95 °C for 45s, 66 °C for 30 s and 72 °C for 45 s and a final extension of 72 °C for 2 min. Negative control reactions were included to access possible PCR reagent contaminations. The final PCR reactions were cleaned up using AMPureXP beads (Beckman Coulter, Brea, CA, USA) and samples were pooled in the sequencing libraries for quantification. The DNA concentration of the pool amplicon was estimated with Picogreen dsDNA assays (Invitrogen, Waltham, MA, USA), and then the pooled libraries were diluted for accurate qPCR quantification using a KAPA Library Quantification Kit for Illumina platforms (KAPA Biosystems, Woburn, MA, USA). The library pool was adjusted to a final concentration of 11.5 pM and sequenced in a MiSeq system, using the standard Illumina primers provided in the kit. A single-end 300nt run was performed using a V2 × 300 sequencing kit. Original sequencing data are available at NCBI BioProject PRJNA546137.

2.3. Microbiome Profile Evaluation Through Bioinformatics Analysis

After the amplicon sequencing, the EncodeTools Metabarcode Pipeline (BiomeHub, Florianópolis, SC, Brazil) was used [27]. In this pipeline, the sequenced reads were quality filtered and primers trimmed resulting in a read of 283pb. Sequence reads smaller than expected, with remaining adapter sequences or more than one mismatch in the primer were excluded. All the reads that passed this quality assessment were clustered into 100% identity oligotypes and analyzed with Deblur [28] and the VSEARCH [29] packages to remove possible erroneous and chimeric reads. Oligotypes below a frequency of 0.2% in the samples were removed. Additionally, a negative control filter was implemented. If any oligotype was observed in the negative controls, it was checked against the samples and removed from the results.

After all, the oligotypes were used for taxonomical assignment with the BLAST [30] tool against a reference genome database constructed with NCBI and *in-house* bacterial genome sequences. Taxonomy was assigned to each oligotype using a lowest common ancestor (LCA) algorithm. If more than one bacterial reference can be assigned to the same oligotype with equivalent similarity and coverage metrics, the EncodeTools Metabarcode Taxonomy Assignment algorithm leads the taxonomy to the lowest level of possible unambiguous resolution (e.g., genus, family, kingdom) according with the similarity thresholds previously stablished [31].

Microbiome data comparison and diversity analysis were conducted inside the R statistical environment (R version 3.6.0). The Phyloseq R package [32] was used for alpha diversity analysis in the plot_richness function. Raw amplicon sequences were used to construct phylogenetic trees using FastTree 2.1 [33] and these were considered to calculate weighted UniFrac distances [34]. Beta diversity analyses used a proportion-normalized abundances [35,36] to calculate Bray–Curtis dissimilarity and weighted UniFrac using the Phyloseq's distance function. Nonparametric tests, including the Kruskall-Wallis and Wilcoxon tests were used as implemented in base R and in coin R package [37].

DESEq2 R package was used to identify differentially abundant genera with the Generalized Linear Model implemented [38]. The obtained *p*-values were corrected according to Benjamini and Hochberg procedure [39]. Values were reported as fold-changes in the log2 scale (log2 FC).

Graphical visualizations for the analysis in the boxplots, principal coordinates analysis (PCoA) and heatmap were generated with the ggplot2 R package [40].

3. Results

Twenty-one patients were included in this study, eleven in the control group and ten in endometriotic group. A total of 47 samples were collected and processed for the evaluation of their bacterial profile: 21 samples of vaginal fluid, 18 eutopic endometrium and 8 endometriotic lesion samples.

Considering all collected samples, we were able to identify 51 different bacterial genera, in a total of 414,787.00 reads, with an average of 8465.04 reads per sample.

Microbiome sequencing from vaginal fluid, eutopic endometrium and endometriotic lesions resulted in similar microorganism profiles, which were composed most abundantly by the bacterial genus *Lactobacillus*, *Gardnerella*, *Streptococcus* and *Prevotella* (Figure 1).

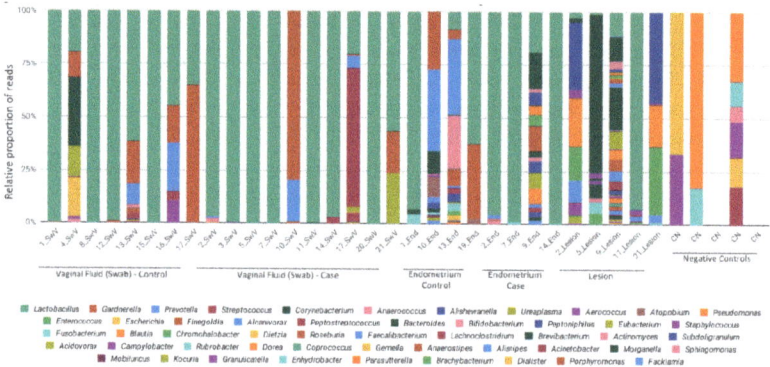

Figure 1. Relative abundance of bacterial profiles. Bacterial composition of each sample is reported by color bars relative to a 100% scale. Results are presented by the taxonomic rank of genus. SwV—vaginal fluid (Swab), End—endometrium, CN—negative controls.

Eutopic endometrium, as well as endometriotic lesion samples, had lower amount of detected relative reads in comparison to vaginal fluid samples (Figure 2), on the other hand, these samples showed less diversity, with which showed a marked predominance of *Lactobacillus*.

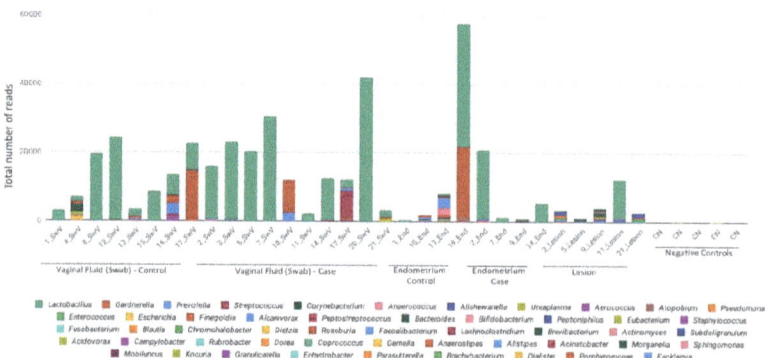

Figure 2. Total reads sequenced for each sample. Bacterial composition of each sample is reported by different color bars and scaled as the total number of reads for each sample. Results are presented by the taxonomic rank of genus. SwV—vaginal fluid (Swab), End—endometrium, CN—negative controls.

We found that endometriotic lesion samples had the most microorganism diversity which included *Lactobacillus, Enterococcus, Gardnerella, Pseudomonas, Alishewanella, Ureaplasma* and *Aerococcus* (Figure 1).

Negative controls (CN) were included in Figures 1 and 2 to demonstrate the lower and different number of reads obtained from kits and reagents background. An average of 66 reads per control was recovered, with a minimum of 45 and a maximum of 204. Negative controls have a totally different bacterial profile from the samples, which demonstrates that there was no contamination of the reagents, and that the presence of microorganisms comes from the studied samples.

A slightly significant difference ($p = 0.036$) among the bacterial composition of lesions (E) compared to other samples was observed when beta-diversity analysis, with weighted UniFrac distances were used, but no differences among samples were observed in Bray-Curtis dissimilarity (Figure 3A).

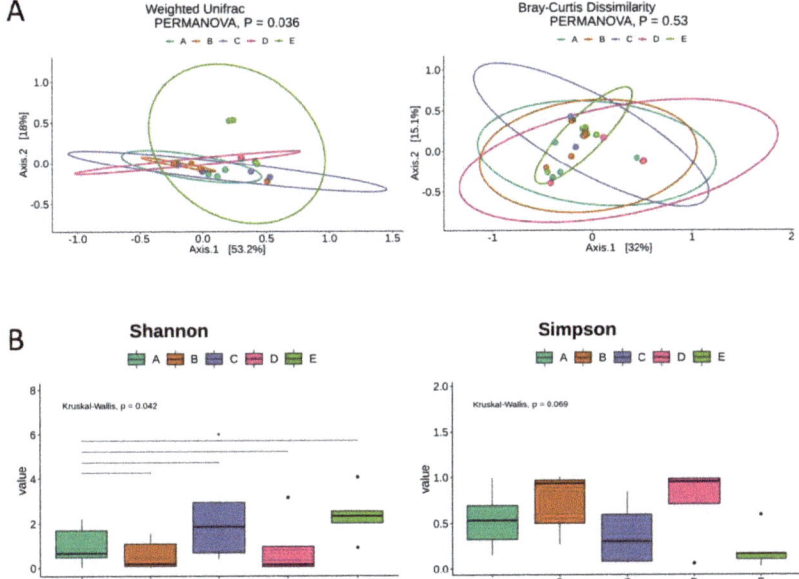

Figure 3. Alpha and beta-diversity analysis. (**A**) Principal coordinates analysis (PCoA) made with weighted UniFrac distances and Bray-Curtis dissimilarity. Sample groups are represented by the letters: A (dark green)-control swab from vaginal fluid; B (orange)-case swab from vaginal fluid; C (purple)-control endometrial tissue; D (pink)-case endometrial tissue; and **E** (light green)-lesion. (**B**) Alpha diversity indexes of Shannon and Simpson are sowed in the boxplots for each collection site group of samples (A, B, C, D and E). Kruskall-Wallis and Wilcoxon tests are showed for group and paired groups comparison, respectively (represented by solid lined above boxplots, only significative comparisons were shown and marked with an *). Black solid points represent outlier samples.

Already when alpha-diversity analysis considering Shannon and Simpson indices was used, we observed highly variable results, but similar diversity levels with the other samples (Figure 3B), despite the tendency to a lower alpha-diversity in endometriotic lesions compared to control vaginal fluid samples.

The most abundant genera detected in the collection sites were plotted (Figure 4A) and it was possible to observe some patterns like the predominance of *Lactobacillus* in vaginal fluid and endometrial samples. The high abundance of *Gardnerella* and *Prevotella* could be observed in the control samples of vaginal fluid and endometrium, while endometriotic lesions showed a higher prevalence of *Alishewanella, Enterococcus* and *Pseudomonas*. This bacterial profile of lesions was also detected in DESeq2 differential abundance analysis, with a significant result (Figure 4B).

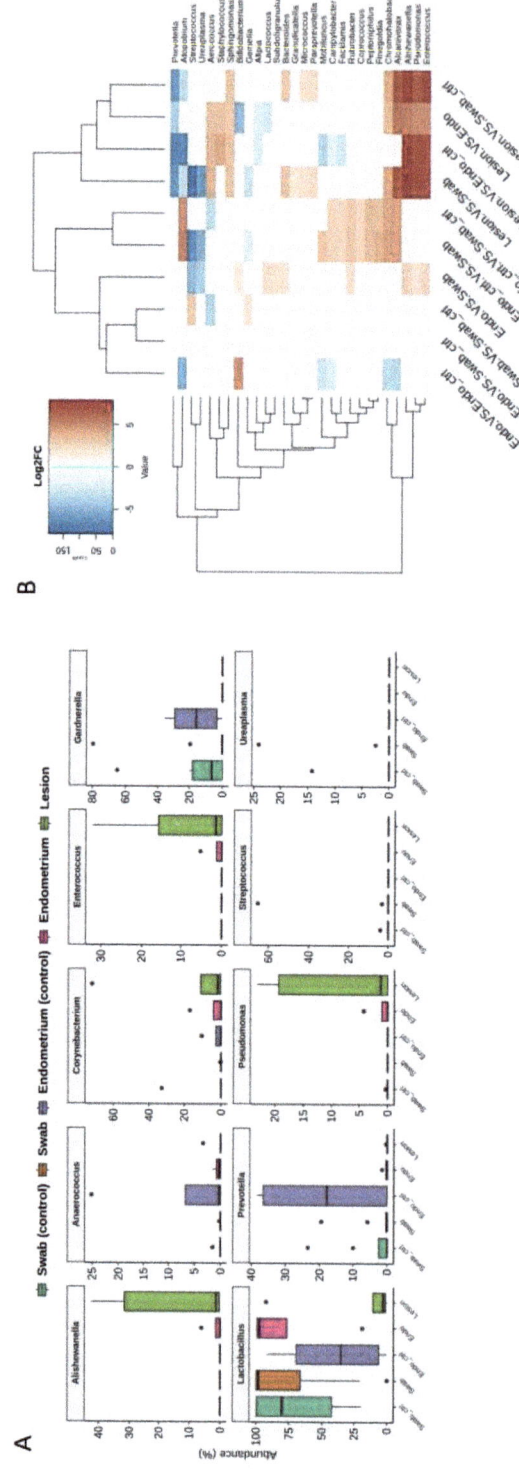

Figure 4. Relative and differential abundances. (**A**) Boxplots represent the most abundant genera detected and their distribution in the samples. Swab_ctrl—control swab from vaginal fluid; Swab—case swab from vaginal fluid; Endo_ctrl—control endometrial tissue; Endo—case endometrial tissue; lesion—samples from endometriosis lesion. Black solid points represent outlier samples for each group. (**B**) Differential abundance heatmap comparing all the collection sites from case and control samples. Results are showed as the log2FC for the differentially detected genera. Most abundant genera are showed as red values considering the first sample category in the bottom legend.

4. Discussion

In this study, we report the microbiome profile from deep endometriotic lesions in Brazilian women.

We detected the presence of microorganisms of the genus *Lactobacillus*, *Enterococcus*, *Gardnerella*, *Pseudomonas*, *Alishewanella*, *Ureaplasma* and *Aerococcus* in deep endometriotic lesions of fifty percent of our endometriosis patient group.

When we compared the microorganism profile from lesions with that found in vaginal fluid and eutopic endometrium of patients with endometriosis, slightly significant differences were found, with a major diversity seen in lesions. Beside this difference, this microbiome data did not reveal a strict bacterial profile specific to the collection sites.

Similar profile between samples derived from 14 women with endometriosis and 14 healthy controls also was observed in a study conduct by Ata et al. [24]. Despite overall similar vaginal, cervical and intestinal microbiota composition between endometriosis and control groups, the authors observed differences at the genus level, with an absence of *Atopobium* in the vaginal and cervical microbiota of the endometriosis group, and enhanced presence of *Gardnerella*, *Streptococcus*, *Escherichia*, *Shigella*, and *Ureaplasma*.

Our results reflect similar profiles of microorganisms as also those obtained by Chen et al. [23] for vaginal and endometrial samples, where the samples collected from endometrium tissue showed a transition profile from the vagina to the upper reproductive tract without sufficient differentiation from other sites of the female reproductive tract. However, the authors still found a change in the microbiota in the peritoneal fluid of women with endometriosis. This alteration found in the peritoneal fluid reinforces our hypothesis that there is an involvement of microorganisms and the immune system in the process of establishment and maintenance of lesions.

Our group investigated the expression of toll-like receptors (TLRs), in T reg cells isolated from peritoneal fluid from patients with and without endometriosis, and we found that there is a change in the activation of TLRs receptors in women with endometriosis, where TLR 1, 2, 3, 4, 5, 6, 7 and 8 were expressed in regulatory T cells isolated from peritoneal fluid from women with endometriosis while only TLR1 and TLR2 receptors were expressed in women without endometriosis [41].

These findings are in line with the findings of this study, which shows that endometriotic lesions have a greater diversity of microorganisms, which consequently cause Treg cells to express a greater number of toll-type receptors, and that there is a relationship between the presence of microorganisms and the inflammatory process.

A retrospective study involving 141.460 patients, out of which 28,292 presented PID (pelvic inflammatory disease) and 113,168 were healthy, showed the correlation between microorganisms and inflammation, suggesting that PID patients were at high risk (three times more) for developing endometriosis than those without PID, suggesting that such bacterial transport in women with PID could facilitate contamination of the upper reproductive tract and pelvic cavity, leading to endometriosis [42]. PID is characterized as a disease caused by the passage of pathogenic bacteria from the vagina to the uterus, fallopian tubes and ovaries.

Present in the plasma membrane or inside vesicles, TLRs are the first receptors to recognize molecular signals of pathogen-associated patterns (PAMPs), triggering a cascade of cellular events. Next, receptors present in the cytosol are activated, via activator protein (AP1) and via interferon regulatory factors (IRFs). These receptors form cytosolic molecular complexes, called inflammasomes, activate caspase- 1 and the production of cytokines, such as IL-1β and IL-18 that induce pyroptosis and apoptosis [43–47]. This process involving TLR receptors, inflammasomes and cytokine production leads to the immune system's response against a wide variety of microorganisms.

These would dampen the natural inflammatory process responsible for the elimination of the retro-flowing uterine endometrial cells during menstruation. As a result, the attachment of ectopic endometrial cells to the peritoneal surfaces would be facilitated. This hypothesis has also been brought forward by other studies related to this topic [48–54].

Our finding of microorganisms in the endometriotic lesions themselves is important as it may advance the hypothesis that one or all of these also ectopically found bacteria may be implicated in the maintenance and survival of the ectopic endometrial cells. The fact that they are also found in the uterine cavity and in the vagina would only be expected.

This was a preliminary evaluation of endometriotic lesions microbiome and there are limitations to the study. A new study with a larger number of patients has to be carried out to confirm the results observed in patients with endometriosis. Moreover, the relation between the presence of these microorganisms and their metabolites in the peritoneal fluid or in the endometriosis lesions should be explored, especially looking into regulation of inflammation and immune responses. As one of the functions of the peritoneal fluid is to remove pathogens the presence of microorganisms in the peritoneal cavity may indicate a poor in situ immune response, one of the possible causes of endometriosis [55].

5. Conclusions

In conclusion, this study revealed that deep endometriotic lesions present a diversity of bacteria as observed in a microbiome analysis using high-throughput DNA sequencing methods. We understand that this result may open new avenues to the study endometriosis and eventually could lead to the development of a noninvasive test for the disease.

Author Contributions: C.H., S.P., A.F.R.S. and L.F.V.d.O. designed the study. C.H., H.M. and S.P. collected the samples. P.S., A.P.C., A.F.R.S. and L.F.V.d.O. conducted the laboratory sample processing. C.H., P.S., A.F.R.S., A.P.C. and L.F.V.d.O. analyzed the results. C.H., S.P., A.F.R.S., P.S. contributed to discussion of results. All authors have read and agree to the published version of the manuscript.

Funding: This research received no external funding.

Conflicts of Interest: The authors declare no conflicts of interest.

References

1. De Paula Andres, M.; Lopes, L.A.; Baracat, E.C.; Podgaec, S. Dienogest in the treatment of endometriosis: Systematic review. *Arch. Gynecol. Obstet.* **2015**, *292*, 523–529. [CrossRef] [PubMed]
2. Parasar, P.; Ozcan, P.; Terry, K.L. Endometriosis: Epidemiology, Diagnosis and Clinical Management. *Curr. Obstet. Gynecol. Rep.* **2017**, *6*, 34–41. [CrossRef] [PubMed]
3. Nisolle, M.; Donnez, J. Peritoneal endometriosis, ovarian endometriosis, and adenomyotic nodules of the rectovaginal septum are three different entities. *Fertil. Steril.* **1997**, *68*, 585–596. [CrossRef]
4. Bassi, M.A.; Arias, V.; D'Amico, N.; Gueuvoghlanian-Silva, B.Y.; Abrao, M.S.; Podgaec, S. Deep Invasive Endometriosis Lesions of the Rectosigmoid May Be Related to Alterations in Cell Kinetics. *Reprod Sci.* **2015**, *22*, 1122–1128. [CrossRef]
5. Santulli, P.; Tran, C.; Gayet, V.; Bourdon, M.; Maignien, L.; Pocate-Cheriet, K.; Chapron, C.; de Ziegler, D. Oligo-anovulation is not a rarer feature in women with documented endometriosis. *Fertil. Steril.* **2018**, *110*, 941–948. [CrossRef]
6. Klemmt, P.A.B.; Starzinski-Powitz, A. Molecular and Cellular Pathogenesis of Endometriosis. *Curr. Womens Health Rev.* **2018**, *14*, 106–116. [CrossRef]
7. Sampson, J.A. Metastatic or Embolic Endometriosis, due to the Menstrual Dissemination of Endometrial Tissue into the Venous Circulation. *Am. J. Pathol.* **1927**, *3*, 93–110.
8. Silvae, J.C.R.; da Fortunato, G.G.; Barbosa, C.P. Aspectos Gerais da Etiopatogenia da Endometriose. In *Coleção Febrasgo Endometriose*, 1st ed.; Podgaec, S., de Janeiro, R., Eds.; Elsevier: Amsterdam, The Netherlands, 2015; pp. 27–34.
9. Zhang, T.; De Carolis, C.; Man, G.C.W.; Wang, C.C. The link between immunity, autoimmunity and endometriosis: A literature update. *Autoimmun. Rev.* **2018**, *17*, 945–955. [CrossRef]
10. Podgaec, S.; junior, J.A.D.; Chapron, C.; de Oliveira, R.M.; Baracat, E.; Abrao, M.S. Th1 and Th2 immune responses related to pelvic endometriosis. *Rev. Assoc. Med. Bras.* **2010**, *56*, 92–98. [CrossRef]
11. Podgaec, S.; Rizzo, L.V.; Fernandes, L.F.; Baracat, E.C.; Abrao, M.S. CD4$^+$ CD25^{high} Foxp3$^+$ cells increased in the peritoneal fluid of patients with endometriosis. *Am. J. Reprod Immunol.* **2012**, *68*, 301–308. [CrossRef]

12. Sourial, S.; Tempest, N.; Hapangama, D.K. Theories on the pathogenesis of endometriosis. *Int. J. Reprod. Med.* **2014**, *2014*, 1–9. [CrossRef] [PubMed]
13. Khan, K.N.; Fujishita, A.; Hiraki, K.; Kitajima, M.; Nakashima, M.; Fushiki, S.; Kitawaki, J. Bacterial contamination hypothesis: A new concept in endometriosis. *Reprod. Med. Biol.* **2018**, *18*, 125–133. [CrossRef] [PubMed]
14. Gueuvoghlanian-Silva, B.Y.; Bellelis, P.; Barbeiro, F.D.; Hernandes, C.; Podgaec, S. Treg and NK cells related cytokines are associated with deep rectosigmoid endometriosis and clinical symptoms related to the disease. *J. Reprod. Immunol.* **2018**, *126*, 32–38. [CrossRef] [PubMed]
15. Bellelis, P.; Barbeiro, D.F.; Gueuvoghlanian-Silva, B.Y.; Kalil, J.; Abrão, M.S.; Podgaec, S. Interleukin-15 and Interleukin-7 are the Major Cytokines to Maintain Endometriosis. *Gynecol. Obstet. Invest.* **2019**, *84*, 435–444. [CrossRef] [PubMed]
16. Akiyama, K.; Nishioka, K.; Khan, K.N.; Tanaka, Y.; Mori, T.; Nakaya, T.; Kitawaki, J. Molecular detection of microbial colonization in cervical mucus of women with and without endometriosis. *Am. J. Reprod. Immunol.* **2019**, *82*, 1–9. [CrossRef] [PubMed]
17. Bullon, P.; Manuel Navarro, J. Inflammasome as a key pathogenic mechanism in endometriosis. *Curr. Drug Targets* **2017**, *18*, 997–1002. [CrossRef] [PubMed]
18. Chadchan, S.B.; Cheng, M.; Parnell, L.A.; Yin, Y.; Schriefer, A.; Mysorekar, I.U.; Kommagani, R. Antibiotic therapy with metronidazole reduces endometriosis disease progression in mice: A potential role for gut microbiota. *Human Reprod.* **2019**, *34*, 1106–1116. [CrossRef]
19. Campos, G.B.; Marques, L.M.; Rezende, I.S. Mycoplasma genitalium can modulate the local immune response in patients with endometriosis. *Fertil. Steril.* **2018**, *109*, 549–560. [CrossRef]
20. Khan, K.N.; Kitajima, M.; Hiraki, K.; Yamaguchi, N.; Katamine, S.; Matsuyama, T.; Nakashima, M.; Fujishita, A.; Ishimaru, T.; Masuzaki, H. Escherichia coli contamination of menstrual blood and effect of bacterial endotoxin on endometriosis. *Fertil. Steril.* **2010**, *94*, 860–863. [CrossRef]
21. Khan, K.N.; Fujishita, A.; Kitajima, M.; Hiraki, K.; Nakashima, M.; Masuzaki, H. Intra-uterine microbial colonization and occurrence of endometritis in women with endometriosis. *Human Reprod.* **2014**, *29*, 2446–2456. [CrossRef]
22. Khan, K.N.; Fujishita, A.; Masumoto, H.; Muto, H.; Kitajima, M.; Masuzaki, H.; Kitawaki, J. Molecular detection of intrauterine microbial colonization in women with endometriosis. *Eur. J. Obstet. Gynecol. Reprod. Biol.* **2016**, *199*, 69–75. [CrossRef] [PubMed]
23. Chen, C.; Song, X.; Wei, W.; Zhong, H.; Dai, J.; Lan, Z. The microbiota continuum along the female reproductive tract and its relation to uterine-related diseases. *Nat. Commun.* **2017**, *17*, 875–878. [CrossRef] [PubMed]
24. Ata, B.; Yildiz, S.; Turkgeldi, E.; Brocal, V.P.; Dinleyici, E.C.; Moya, A.; Urman, B. The Endobiota Study: Comparison of Vaginal, Cervical and Gut Microbiota between Women with Stage 3/4 Endometriosis and Healthy Controls. *Sci. Rep.* **2019**, *9*, 2204. [CrossRef] [PubMed]
25. Wang, Y.; Qian, P. Conservative Fragments in Bacterial 16S rRNA Genes and Primer Design for 16S Ribosomal DNA Amplicons in Metagenomic Studies. *PLoS ONE* **2009**, *4*, e7401. [CrossRef]
26. Caporaso, J.G.; Christian, L.L.; Walters, W.A.; Berg-lyons, D.; Huntley, J.; Fierer, N.; Owens, S.; Betley, J.; Fraser, L.; Bauer, M.; et al. Ultra-high-throughput microbial community analysis on the Illumina HiSeq and MiSeq platforms. *ISME J.* **2012**, *6*, 1621–1624. [CrossRef] [PubMed]
27. Christoff, A.P.; Cruz, G.F.N.; Sereia, A.F.R.; Yamanaka, L.E.; Silveira, P.P.; Oliveira, L.F.V. End-to-end assessment of fecal bacteriome analysis: From sample processing to DNA sequencing and bioinformatics results. *bioRxiv* **2019**, 646349. [CrossRef]
28. Amir, A.; McDonald, D.; Navas-Molina, J.A.; Kopylova, E.; Morton, J.T.; Xu, Z.Z.; Kightley, E.P.; Thompson, L.R.; Hyde, E.R.; Gonzalez, A.; et al. Deblur Rapidly Resolves Single-Nucleotide Community Sequence Patterns. *mSystems* **2017**, *2*, e00191-16. [CrossRef]
29. Rognes, T.; Flouri, T.; Nichols, B.; Quince, C.; Mahé, F. VSEARCH: A versatile open source tool for metagenomics. *PeerJ* **2016**, *4*, e2584. [CrossRef]
30. Altschul, S.; Gish, W.; Miller, W.; Myers, E.; Lipman, D. Basic local alignment search tool. *J. Mol. Biol.* **1990**, *215*, 403–410. [CrossRef]

31. Yarza, P.; Yilmaz, P.; Pruesse, E.; Glöckner, F.O.; Ludwig, W.; Schleifer, K.H.; Whitman, W.B.; Euzéby, J.; Amann, R.; Rosselló-Móra, R. Uniting the classification of cultured and uncultured bacteria and archaea using 16S rRNA gene sequences. *Nat. Rev. Microbiol.* **2014**, *2*, 635–645. [CrossRef]
32. McMurdie, P.; Holmes, S. Phyloseq: An R Package for Reproducible Interactive Analysis and Graphics of Microbiome Census Data. *PLoS ONE* **2013**, *8*, e61217. [CrossRef] [PubMed]
33. Price, M.; Dehal, P.; Arkin, A. FastTree 2—Approximately Maximum-Likelihood Trees for Large Alignments. *PLoS ONE* **2010**, *5*, e9490. [CrossRef] [PubMed]
34. Lozupone, C.; Knight, R. UniFrac: A New Phylogenetic Method for Comparing Microbial Communities. *Appl. Environ. Microbiol.* **2015**, *71*, 8228. [CrossRef] [PubMed]
35. Weiss, S.; Xu, Z.Z.; Peddada, S.; Amir, A.; Bittinger, K.; Gonzalez, A.; Lozupone, C.; Zaneveld, J.R.; Vázquez-Baeza, Y.; Birmingham, A.; et al. Normalization and microbial differential abundance strategies depend upon data characteristics. *Microbiome* **2017**, *5*, 27. [CrossRef]
36. McMurdie, P.; Holmes, S. Waste Not, Want Not: Why Rarefying Microbiome Data Is Inadmissible. *PLoS Comput. Biol.* **2014**, *10*, e1003531. [CrossRef]
37. Hothorn, T.; Hornik, K.; Wiel, M.A.; Zeileis, A. Implementing a class of permutation tests: The coin package. *J. Stat. Softw.* **2008**, *28*, 23. [CrossRef]
38. Love, M.; Huber, W.; Anders, S. Moderated estimation of fold change and dispersion for RNA-seq data with DESeq2. *Genome Biol.* **2014**, *15*, 550. [CrossRef]
39. Benjamini, Y.; Hochberg, Y. Controlling the false discovery rate: A practical and powerful approach to multiple hypothesis testing. *J. R. Stat. Soc. B* **1995**, *57*, 289–300. [CrossRef]
40. Wickham, H. *ggplot2: Elegant Graphics for Data Analysis*; Springer: Berlin/Heidelberg, Germany, 2016.
41. Hernandes, C.; Gueuvoghlanian-Silva, B.Y.; Monnaka, V.U.; Ribeiro, N.M.; Pereira, W.O.; Podgaec, S. Regulatory T cells isolated from endometriotic peritoneal fluid express a different number of Toll-like receptors expressed. *Einstein (São Paulo)* **2020**, *18*, eAO5294.
42. Tai, F.W.; Chang, C.Y.; Chiang, J.H.; Lin, W.C.; Wan, L. Association of Pelvic Inflammatory Disease with Risk of Endometriosis: A Nationwide Cohort Study Involving 141,460 Individuals. *J. Clin. Med.* **2018**, *7*, 379. [CrossRef]
43. Kawai, T.; Akira, S. The roles of TLRs, RLRs and NLRs in pathogen recognition. *Int. Immunol.* **2009**, *21*, 317–337. [CrossRef] [PubMed]
44. Lamkanfi, M.; Dixit, V.M. Mechanisms and functions of inflammasomes. *Cell* **2014**, *15*, 1013–1022. [CrossRef] [PubMed]
45. Broz, P.; Dixit, V.M. Inflammasomes: Mechanism of assembly, regulation and signalling. *Nat. Rev. Immunol.* **2016**, *16*, 407. [CrossRef] [PubMed]
46. Sharma, D.; Kanneganti, T.D. The cell biology of inflammasomes: Mechanisms of inflammasome activation and regulation. *J. Cell Biol.* **2016**, *213*, 617–629. [CrossRef] [PubMed]
47. Webster, S.J.; Goodall, J.C. New concepts in Chlamydia induced inflammasome responses. *Microb. Infect.* **2018**, *20*, 424–431. [CrossRef] [PubMed]
48. Caramalho, I.; Lopes-Carvalho, T.; Ostler, D.; Zelenay, S.; Haury, M.; Demengeot, J. Regulatory T cells selectively express toll-like receptors and are activated by lipopolysaccharide. *J. Exp. Med.* **2003**, *197*, 403–411. [CrossRef] [PubMed]
49. Netea, M.G.; Sutmuller, R.; Hermann, C.; Van der Graaf, C.A.; Van der Meer, J.W.; Van Krieken, J.H.; Hartung, T.; Adema, G.; Kullberg, B.J. Toll-like receptor 2 suppresses immunity against Candida albicans through induction of IL-10 and regulatory T cells. *J. Immunol.* **2004**, *172*, 3712–3718. [CrossRef]
50. Peng, G.; Guo, Z.; Kiniwa, Y.; Voo, K.S.; Peng, W.; Fu, T.; Wang, D.Y.; Li, Y.; Wang, H.Y. Toll-like receptor 8-mediated reversal of CD4+ regulatory T cell function. *Science* **2005**, *309*, 1380–1384. [CrossRef]
51. Liu, G.; Zhao, Y. Toll-like receptors and immune regulation: Their direct and indirect modulation on regulatory CD4+ CD25+ T cells. *Immunology* **2007**, *122*, 149–156. [CrossRef]
52. Van Maren, W.W.; Jacobs, J.F.; de Vries, I.J.; Nierkens, S.; Adema, G.J. Toll-like receptor signalling on Tregs: To suppress or not to suppress? *Immunology* **2008**, *124*, 445–452. [CrossRef]
53. Olivier, A.; Dong, H.; Sparwasser, T.; Majilessi, L.; Leclerc, C. The adjuvant effect of TLR agonists on CD4+ effector T cells is under the indirect control of regulatory T cells. *Eur. J. Immunol.* **2011**, *41*, 2303–2313. [CrossRef] [PubMed]

54. de Barros, I.B.L.; Malvezzi, H.; Gueuvoghlanian-Silva, B.Y.; Piccinato, C.A.; Rizzo, L.V.; Podgaec, S. Corrigendum to "What do we know about regulatory T cells and endometriosis? A systematic review". *J. Reprod. Immunol.* **2017**, *121*, 48–55. [CrossRef] [PubMed]
55. Capobianco, A.; Cottone, L.; Monno, A.; Manfredi, A.A.; Rovere-Querini, P. The peritoneum: Healing, immunity, and diseases. *J. Pathol.* **2017**, *243*, 137–147. [CrossRef] [PubMed]

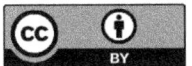
© 2020 by the authors. Licensee MDPI, Basel, Switzerland. This article is an open access article distributed under the terms and conditions of the Creative Commons Attribution (CC BY) license (http://creativecommons.org/licenses/by/4.0/).

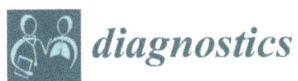

Review

Endometriosis in Menopause—Renewed Attention on a Controversial Disease

Cristina Secosan [1], Ligia Balulescu [1,*], Simona Brasoveanu [1], Oana Balint [1], Paul Pirtea [2], Grigoraş Dorin [1] and Laurentiu Pirtea [1]

1. Department of Obstetrics and Gynecology, University of Medicine and Pharmacy "Victor Babeş", 300041 Timişoara, Romania; cristina.secosan@gmail.com (C.S.); brasoveanu_simona@yahoo.com (S.B.); oana.balint@gmail.com (O.B.); grigorasdorin@ymail.com (G.D.); laurentiupirtea@gmail.com (L.P.)
2. Department of Ob Gyn and Reproductive Medicine, Hopital Foch—Faculté de Medicine Paris Ouest (UVSQ), 92151 Suresnes, France; paulpirtea@gmail.com
* Correspondence: ligia_balulescu@yahoo.com

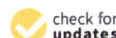

Received: 13 January 2020; Accepted: 27 February 2020; Published: 29 February 2020

Abstract: Endometriosis, an estrogen-dependent inflammatory disease characterized by the ectopic presence of endometrial tissue, has been the topic of renewed research and debate in recent years. The paradigm shift from the belief that endometriosis only affects women of reproductive age has drawn attention to endometriosis in both premenarchal and postmenopausal patients. There is still scarce information in literature regarding postmenopausal endometriosis, the mostly studied and reported being the prevalence in postmenopausal women. Yet, other important issues also need to be addressed concerning diagnosis, pathophysiology, and management. We aimed at summarizing the currently available data in literature in order to provide a concise and precise update regarding information available on postmenopausal endometriosis.

Keywords: endometriosis; menopause; diagnosis; management; malignancy

1. Introduction

The concept that endometriosis is a disease that only affects women of reproductive age has prevailed since 1942, when the first case of endometriosis in a postmenopausal patient was reported by Edgar Haydon [1].

In spite of this early report, endometriosis has also been described in premenarchal patients and is a common occurrence in adolescents [2–4].

The recurrence of endometriosis lesions in patients with a prior diagnosis of endometriosis during the premenopausal period or the de novo appearance of endometriosis in postmenopausal patients with no prior history of endometriosis-related complaints has been however well documented in numerous case series, case reports, and retrospective studies [5–9].

The management of endometriosis in postmenopause and hormone replacement therapy (HRT) in patients with a history of endometriosis remains controversial.

2. Prevalence

The incidence of postmenopausal endometriosis reported in literature is of approximately 2–5%. It commonly represents a side effect of HRT, rarely occurring in patients without a history of HRT or Tamoxifen treatment [10]. In a few cases, postmenopausal endometriosis has been described in women who had no history of endometriosis on imaging or surgery prior to menopause [11].

In order to evaluate the prevalence of postmenopausal endometriosis, Haas et al. performed a retrospective epidemiological study on 42,079 women admitted for surgical treatment with histologically confirmed endometriosis. Patients were sorted in 5 years age groups and also in premenopausal, perimenopausal, and postmenopausal subgroups. The results showed that 33,814 patients (80.36%) were in the premenopausal group (age 0–45 years), with 23 patients (0.05%) being younger than 15 years; of the remaining patients, 7191 (17.09%) were in the perimenopausal (45–55 years), and 1074 patients (2.55%) in the postmenopausal group, respectively [6].

3. Pathophysiology

Endometriosis is an estrogen-dependent inflammatory disease characterized by the presence of ectopic endometrial tissue. The pathogenesis of endometriosis remains enigmatic [12].

Postmenopausal endometriosis is considered to have an even more complex pathophysiology than premenopausal endometriosis. It is still unclear whether this represents a recurrence or continuation of a previous disease or a de novo condition. Excess estrogen, in general, represents a promoting factor for endometriosis. The arrest of estrogen production at the level of the ovaries at the time of menopause is counterbalanced by peripheral estrogen production from conversion of androgens (especially in the adipose tissue and skin). The leading estrogen found in these patients is estrone.

An attractive theory regarding the pathogenic mechanism of postmenopausal endometriosis involves the "estrogen threshold", i.e., when a certain estrogen level is reached or surpassed in postmenopausal patients it activates undetected or "transient" foci of endometriosis.

In addition to the peripheral estrogen production, a high circulating level of estrogen may be of external source, especially in the form of phytoestrogens and HRT. Phytoestrogens appear to exert estrogenic effects on the uterus, breast, and pituitary and could also support the growth of endometriotic lesions [13–15].

Despite the fact that postmenopausal endometriosis has the same immunochemical profile as premenopausal endometriosis and has the potential to reactivate under estrogen stimulation, endometriosis lesions in the postmenopausal period seem to be less common, less extensive, and less active in most cases [16].

4. Symptomatology

The clinical presentation of endometriosis in menopausal patients is unspecific, such as pelvic pain, ovarian cysts, or intestinal symptoms. Given the age of the patients, they are often suspected of a neoplastic process. As a general consideration, all postmenopausal patients should be evaluated for malignancy if a new suspicious structure is found on ultrasound examination.

In menopausal women with a history of endometriosis, the drop in estrogen levels after menopause relieves the endometriosis-related symptoms but generates specific menopausal ones, such as mood swings, hot flushes, vaginal atrophy, and night sweats [5,17]. The clinical grim reality is that the severity of the disease is not necessarily reflected in the degree of discomfort. Commonly, the complaints of pelvic pain underestimate the disease's severity in both premenopausal and postmenopausal endometriosis.

5. Diagnosis

Despite intensive research conducted in the last decades, endometriosis remains a disease with a delayed diagnosis, especially in older patients. This results from the lack of noninvasive tools available for early stage diagnosis. For many years, there has been a long-standing myth that endometriosis is a disease that affects only adult women of reproductive age. However, in recent years, focus has turned to the diagnosis of endometriosis in postmenopausal patients, given that the onset of pain can start after the onset of menopause, with reports of endometriosis occurring even in 80-year-old patients [1,5].

The ovaries are the most common location of endometriotic lesions in postmenopausal patients (79.2% of cases) [18].

Distinction between endometriosis lesions and cancer is complicated by the fact that some of the risk factors are similar, such as low parity rate, infertility, late childbearing age, and a short duration of oral contraceptive use [19].

Currently, laparoscopy and biopsy for histological confirmation of suspicious lesions is the gold standard for diagnosis of endometriosis, irrespective of age. Laparoscopy, the standard technique for inspecting the pelvis, can provide simultaneous diagnosis and treatment of lesions. Additional tools are needed for a noninvasive diagnostic and classification. To this date, no serum marker or test is available for reliably diagnosing endometriosis [20,21]. Regarding imaging investigations, MRI and ultrasound are important, but findings are more difficult to interpret in menopausal patients than in younger patients due to the higher suspicion for neoplastic lesions and the polymorphic aspect of endometriosis.

5.1. Clinical Examination

The patient's medical history, clinical examination, or preoperative symptoms have a limited role in determining the extent of endometriosis lesions as there is no direct relationship between symptoms and the anatomic-surgical characteristics of endometriotic lesions [22]. Also, there is usually a discrepancy between the severity of symptoms and the extent of lesions with many patients whose severe lesions remain asymptomatic. This is an important factor contributing to a delay of approximately 6 to 8 years from onset of symptoms to diagnosis in premenopausal and postmenopausal patients alike [23].

Pelvic vaginal and rectal examination is useful in identifying endometriosis nodules in the lower posterior compartment, but clinical examination may be normal in many patients with deep infiltrating endometriosis [23].

5.2. Imaging

While diagnostic laparoscopy remains the gold standard, it is often not the first line of diagnosis any more, as noninvasive testing for early diagnosis and progression of endometriosis is being preferred [24]. Yet, no imaging method can definitively confirm the diagnosis of endometriosis, being notably inconclusive in case of peritoneal implants [25].

Deep infiltrating endometriosis (DIE) can be investigated through several imaging techniques, including transvaginal sonography (TVS), magnetic resonance imaging (MRI), computerized tomography, rectal endoscopic sonography, and three-dimensional (3D) ultrasound [23].

TVS has gained interest in recent years and is starting to be recommended as the first-line investigation technique in endometriosis because it allows extensive exploration of the pelvis, is widely available, cost efficient, and well tolerated [26–28].

TVS has the benefit of a lack of exposure to radiation and is the main method for the evaluation of adnexal masses, but remains limited for the diagnosis of other kinds of endometriosis. Endometriomas have distinct characteristics on ultrasound: unilocular cysts, most often of homogenous "ground glass" appearance. The identification of an endometrioma should alert the clinician to the possibility of moderate-to-advanced stage disease. An important exception is postmenopausal women, in whom ovarian cysts with a "ground glass" appearance are associated with a 44% risk of malignancy. In addition, TVS may have a role in assessing disease involving the bladder and rectum [29].

Computed tomography (CT) plays a major role in the diagnosis of bowel endometriosis in the presence of colon distension. Genitourinary tract involvement should be taken into consideration in case of hydronephrosis or hydroureter diagnosed on CT scan, especially in patients with a history of chronic pelvic pain or in patients with a history of endometriosis. Radiation exposure should be taken into consideration [29].

MRI is a noninvasive diagnostic method of DIE that offers the possibility to fully investigate the pelvic cavity with a high accuracy, but increased costs [30]. Nevertheless, MRI has limited indication in the diagnosis of endometriosis. It can confirm the diagnosis of endometrioma in the presence of an adnexal mass when TVS is uncertain. MRI can also be used as an investigation method when involvement of the ureter is suspected, and may be beneficial in the evaluation of anatomy when expanded pelvic adhesions are suspected [29].

Sonovaginography using saline solution (saline contrast sonovaginography (SCSV)) or gel infusion sonovaginography is a new diagnostic method in DIE. First described by Dessole et al., it consists of TVS combined with the introduction of saline solution or gel infusion into the vagina, which offers the benefit of a more complete view of the vaginal walls and fornix, pouch Douglas, uterosacral ligaments, and rectovaginal septum [22]. The data available in literature is limited, with only a few reports from Brazil, Italy, Romania, and Australia, but the methods seems beneficial in the diagnosis of posterior deep infiltrating endometriosis. Up to date, no studies have reported its use in postmenopausal patients [22,31–33].

The role of double-contrast barium enema (DCBE) in the evaluation of rectovaginal endometriosis is controversial. Some studies have reported high accuracy in predicting the need for intestinal surgery in endometriosis cases. The superiority of DCBE over rectal ultrasound or MRI is not well established, the results reported in literature being scarce and contradictory. However, certain studies have demonstrated a lower sensitivity of DCBE for rectovaginal disease. DCBE does not allow the examination of the entire intestinal wall thickness and does not provide information regarding the depth of infiltration, but may provide useful information for preoperative planning when severe disease is suspected [29].

5.3. Biomarkers

To this date, no specific markers for the diagnosis of endometriosis have been identified. A change in levels of proteins, microRNAs, and other markers corresponding to a disease state could be the basis for identifying novel biomarkers. Endometriosis patients often show modified ranges of CA-125 (Cancer Antigen 125), cytokines, angiogenic and growth factors compared with normal women, but all of these biomarkers are frequently encountered in various other pathologies and are not specific enough for diagnosing endometriosis. A combination of biomarkers may improve the sensitivity and specificity over single biomarker measurements. Moreover, stem cell, proteomic, and genomic studies could contribute to the development of new high-sensitivity biomarkers in the diagnosis of endometriosis in the future [24].

Many authors have studied the role of biomarkers for diagnosis of endometriosis and concluded that, to date, endometrial tissue, menstrual or uterine fluids, and immunologic markers in blood or urine are not recommended for clinical use for diagnosis of endometriosis [24].

Regarding the differential diagnosis between endometriomas and malignant ovarian tumors in postmenopausal patients, we have not found any information in the literature that supports the use of any novel tests, such as OVA1 (Ovarian Malignancy Algorithm), ROMA (risk of ovarian malignancy algorithm), circulating miRs, etc. Despite the potential clinical utility of these biomarkers in the diagnosis of malignant ovarian tumors in premenopausal patients, the costs implied, the lack of easy availability, and the decreased incidence of endometriomas in older patients make the usefulness of novel biomarkers difficult to assess [34–36].

5.4. Minimally Invasive Surgery: Laparoscopy and Robot Assistance

Because of the lack of specific and efficient noninvasive tests for endometriosis, there is often a significant delay in diagnosis of this disease, especially in older patients. The gold standard for the diagnosis of endometriosis remains visual inspection by laparoscopy, preferably with histological confirmation. A positive histological examination confirms the diagnosis, but negative histology does not exclude it, in the presence of pathognomonic lesions [23].

Whether histology should be obtained if peritoneal disease alone is present is controversial: a visual inspection of the pelvis should be enough, but histological confirmation of at least one lesion is ideal. In some cases, histology should be obtained to identify endometriosis and to exclude malignant disease. For example, in ovarian endometriomas (>3 cm in diameter) and in deeply infiltrating disease, a histological confirmation to exclude a rare instance of malignancy is necessary [37].

Laparoscopy is used for the diagnosis and treatment of DIE and serves to eradicate all visible endometriosis implants, especially in postmenopausal patients due to the risk of malignant transformation. Several studies have shown a significant improvement of symptoms and a decreased risk of malignancy in postmenopausal women after complete resection of all visible lesions. Precise preoperative imaging may help guide surgical therapeutic approaches and aid to obtain the best postoperative results [23]. In the last years, the da Vinci surgical system started to be used in the diagnosis and treatment of endometriosis. Three-dimensional (3D) vision offers the advantage of improved depth perception and accuracy in the performance of robotic surgery, particularly for complex surgical tasks such as identifying suspected implants. However, the robotic platform has the distinct disadvantage of offering only a unidirectional view within the abdominal cavity. Authors recommend for the first instance to undertake a diagnostic laparoscopy to exclude a suspected lesion of endometriosis in the upper abdomen, liver, diaphragm, and appendix before using the da Vinci robotic system in the pelvis. Another disadvantage is the loss of haptic feedback to identify fibrotic lesions which are characteristic of deeply infiltrating disease. However, the da Vinci robot may offer improved ease by avoiding hand and more instinctual movement of the wristed instruments in the treatment of endometriosis. The cost related to the procedure also make it unavailable at a large scale [29].

6. Management

6.1. The Impact of Hormone Replacement Therapy in Women with a History of Endometriosis

The recently published guidelines on menopause management have no statements of endometriosis symptoms [38]. The use of HRT raises concerns about disease reactivation and recurrence of pain and need for surgical treatment, and even malignant transformation of residual endometriosis. The risk of recurrence with HRT is considered to be linked to residual disease after surgery. The data regarding hormone therapy regimens is scarce. Continuous combined estrogen–progesterone treatment or tibolone, in patients with or without hysterectomy, is considered to carry a lower risk of disease recurrence, compared with estrogen-only regimens, but larger studies are required in order to prove the safety and efficacy. Management of potential recurrence is best monitored by awareness of the possibility of symptom recurrence. Patients with contraindication or who refuse hormonal treatment should be offered alternative pharmacological treatment for menopausal symptoms and for skeletal protection, if indicated. Herbal products should be avoided as some may contain estrogenic compounds and their efficacy is uncertain [39–41]. The risk of malignant transformation of endometriosis in women with a history of endometriosis who received HRT remains a matter of debate. Long-term follow-up studies are needed to evaluate the risk of an adverse outcome. Further studies are mandatory in order to determine the optimal management of menopause in women with endometriosis [15].

6.2. The Management of De Novo Endometriosis in Postmenopausal Patients and Pain Management

"De novo" endometriosis appears especially after unopposed estrogen therapy or obesity, which has an additional effect for increasing the risk of endometriosis development.

Postmenopausal women with symptomatic endometriosis should be managed surgically with removal of all visible endometriotic tissue because of the higher risk of recurrence and the risk of malignancy [41]. A similar approach is recommended by current ESHRE (European Society of Human Reproduction and Embryology) recommendations. Medical therapy can be used in case of pain recurrence after surgery or if surgery is contraindicated. Co-morbidities represent an additional risk to contraindicate surgery and include advanced age or pelvic adhesions from previous surgery [38,41]. Approximately 12% of all endometriosis cases will finally require a hysterectomy with or without oophorectomy [42,43]. To prevent recurrences, to restore bowel, urinary, or sexual function or to alleviate pain it is now recommended to remove all the implants [38].

Progesterone administration (oral or intrauterine system) has been proposed as a reliable alternative treatment in patients with contraindication for surgery, but, up to date, no extensive data is available and further studies are needed regarding progesterone use in postmenopausal endometriosis [44,45].

Aromatase inhibitors act by decreasing extra-ovarian estrogen production and by blocking the feed-forward stimulation loop between inflammation and aromatase within endometriosis lesions. Only six case reports of aromatase inhibitors administration in postmenopausal patients with a history of endometriosis have been published so far. In 1998, Kayama presented a 57-year-old patient who had presented with recurrent endometriosis with a painful vaginal polypoid mass. The use of Anastrozole reduced the volume of the vaginal mass. Other studies concluded that Letrozole has a similar efficacy to Anastrozole [46–48]. The most important risk of this treatment is osteoporosis and related fractures. Aromatase inhibitors impair bone mineral density and need to be associated with bisphosphonate therapy.

7. Tamoxifen and Postmenopausal Endometriosis

Tamoxifen represents a hormonal substitution therapy used in postmenopausal women with breast cancer. Tamoxifen has antiestrogenic effects on breast tissues but promotes endometriosis through unknown mechanisms. In 1993, the first case of tamoxifen-related endometriosis was reported in a woman who received tamoxifen for 2 years due to breast cancer [49]. In the next year, it was reported another case of operated breast cancer and adjuvant tamoxifen [50]. During the next years, many authors reported cases of ovarian and endometrioid carcinoma in the women who had used tamoxifen [51–54]. Considering that there is no significant statistical evidence, the relation between tamoxifen and malignant transformation may be coincidental [43].

8. Risk of Malignant Transformation

The possible transformation of endometriosis lesions into malignant lesions and their dissemination in the ovaries, bowel, and even lungs has been described. The risk of malignant transformation of endometrioma into an ovarian cancer is estimated at 2% or 3% [41,55], and may be higher in patients receiving estrogen therapy. Furthermore, patients with endometriosis have an increased risk of other malignancies, apart from ovarian cancer [41].

Differential diagnosis of benign from malignant tumors in postmenopausal women is difficult. We must take into account that some endometriosis lesions may have a similar appearance to malignant disease and can cause local and distant metastases and can infiltrate adjacent tissues and organs. Age is an important risk factor for many malignancies, thus it may be questioned whether the postmenopausal endometriosis increases the risk for malignancy [41].

In 1997, Brinton et al. showed that patients with endometriosis seem to have an increased overall cancer risk [56]. Some authors indicate an increased risk of ovarian cancer, calculated to be around 35% for clear cell carcinoma and 19% for endometrioid type carcinoma in women with endometriosis [57].

On the other hand, Somigliana et al. concluded that there is evidence to support that endometriosis should be considered a medical condition associated with a clinically relevant risk of any specific cancer [58].

Regarding the relationship between endometriosis and breast cancer, Bertelsen et al. published a study which followed around 115,000 Danish women over a period of 30 years. Authors concluded that the risk for breast cancer increased with age (<40 years) at diagnosis of endometriosis and it is around 0.97%. The increased risk associated with endometriosis among postmenopausal women may be due to common risk factors between postmenopausal endometriosis and breast cancer or an altered endogenous estrogen [59].

Because endometriosis and ovarian malignancy have some common risk factors, including low parity rate, infertility, late childbearing age, and short duration of oral contraceptive use, in clinical practice is very difficult to discriminate a benign from a malignant tumor in postmenopausal women [60].

In postmenopausal women who underwent surgery for endometriosis, hormonal therapy remains controversial. Unopposed estrogen stimulation is associated with an increased risk of endometrial cancer. Some studies show that exogenous estrogens are increasing the risk of malignancy transformation of endometriosis lesions. In a retrospective study which followed 31 women with cancer developing from endometriosis, Zanetta et al. concluded that prevalence of endometriosis associated with co-existing risk factors (obesity and unopposed estrogen therapy) represents a significant risk factor for the development of cancer in endometriotic lesions [61].

The indication for initiating hormone therapy in women with endometriosis must be carefully evaluated. In premenopausal women who underwent total hysterectomy and bilateral salpingo-oophorectomy due to endometriosis, the benefits of hormone therapy outweigh the risks. Postmenopausal hormone therapy may increase the risk of malignant transformation or recurrence of endometriosis [41,62]. More data are needed to confirm this.

9. Extrapelvic Endometriosis

Extrapelvic endometriosis is a rare clinical condition in postmenopausal women. It affects a slightly older population due to the fact that it takes several years for pelvic endometriosis to metastasize outside the pelvis. Statistical data regarding menopausal patients are limited. The most common location of extrapelvic endometriosis is the gastrointestinal tract, followed by the urinary system. Bladder and ureteral endometriosis are the most common sites for urinary tract involvement [63]. Regarding the gastrointestinal tract, the sigmoid colon is the most commonly involved, followed by the rectum, ileum, appendix, and caecum [64,65]. Extremely rare locations that have been reported include the gallbladder, the Meckel diverticulum, stomach, and endometriosis cysts of the pancreas and liver [63].

Flyckt et al. presented a 59-year-old woman with a periaortic mass with ureteral obstruction. A computed tomography was performed, and a surgical management was necessary to resect the mass. The pathology exam confirmed endometriosis invasion of the inferior vena cava [66].

9.1. Gastrointestinal Tract Endometriosis

In postmenopausal women with low estrogen levels, a vascular transport or metaplasia of intestinal tissue should be considered for the etiology of gastrointestinal tract endometriosis [65]. The intestinal involvement in endometriosis after menopause is a rare phenomenon and it has been described in literature only in case reports (Figure 1).

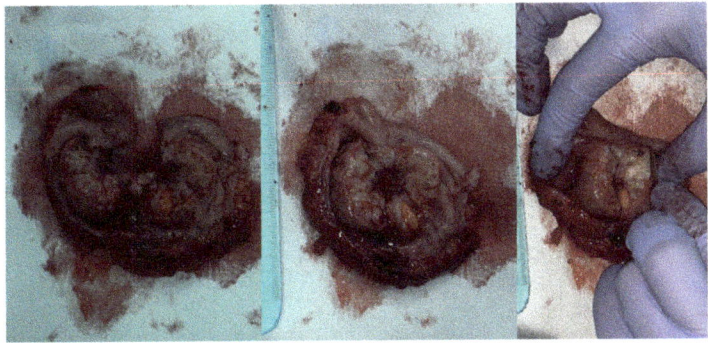

Figure 1. Sigmoid colon endometriosis—macroscopic aspect of the piece after laparoscopic resection using a circular stapler (personal collection, L. Pirtea).

Snyder et al. presented the case of a woman with iron-deficiency anemia, who underwent total hysterectomy with bilateral salpingo-oophorectomy. During the surgical procedure, an endometrial implant at the hepatic flexure was discovered, a rare location for endometriosis. The patient was treated with conjugated estrogen–bazedoxifen to antagonize the effects of estrogen. No evidence of lesion was found at colonoscopy after five months of therapy [11].

Popoutchi reported a rare case of postmenopausal intestinal endometriosis simulating a malignant lesion in a woman who previously underwent hysterectomy with bilateral salpingo-oophorectomy, with no hormone replacement treatment. She was treated by rectosigmoidectomy with colostomy [65].

It is difficult to diagnose bowel endometriosis by colonoscopy because most cases do not infiltrate beyond the serosa and very few infiltrate the mucosa [67]. Deep endometriosis is a very complicated disease to diagnose and treat, especially in older patients [43,68].

Jones et al. reported a case of a surgical menopause for deep rectovaginal endometriosis, with estrogen replacement therapy. A polyp was detected on colonoscopy and the biopsy confirmed a malignant transformation of endometriosis to adenocarcinoma [69].

9.2. Urinary Tract Endometriosis

Urinary tract endometriosis is an uncommon pathology and a silent cause of monolateral or bilateral kidney dysfunction. The diagnosis of urinary tract endometriosis is difficult since the disease is associated with nonspecific symptoms, regardless of the hormonal status [70] (Figure 2).

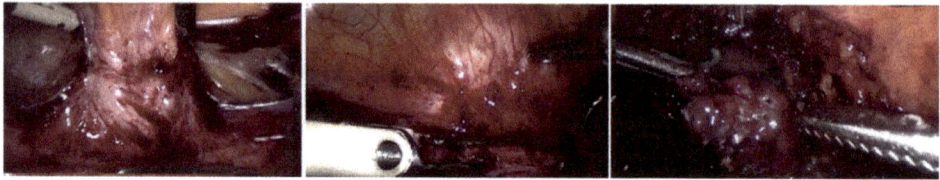

Figure 2. Urinary tract endometriosis—laparoscopic resection of a bladder endometriosis nodule infiltrating the bladder mucosa (personal collection, L. Pirtea).

A few case reports have been published regarding bladder endometriosis in postmenopausal women. Stewart reported a case of bladder endometriosis extending into the bowel in a postmenopausal woman. He concluded that it was due to reactivation of the endometrial implants under exogenous estrogen stimulation [71]. Also, a case of a 68-year-old postmenopausal woman, with no exogenous estrogen therapy, with an abnormal mass of the bladder that turned out to be an endometriosis lesion, was reported. This case suggests that endometriosis may persist even after years of a hormonally castrated state [72].

10. Conclusions

The paradigm shift from the belief that endometriosis only affects women of reproductive age has drawn attention to endometriosis in both premenarchal and postmenopausal patients. Despite its relatively low incidence, physicians should consider endometriosis in cases of unclear pelvic pain in postmenopausal patients, even if the patient has no prior history of endometriosis lesions.

Postmenopausal endometriosis seems to expose the patient to a higher risk of malignant transformation. Due to the lack of high-quality studies, it remains unclear how to advise women with a history of endometriosis regarding the management of menopausal symptoms. The absolute risk of disease recurrence and malignant transformation cannot be quantified, and the impact of HRT use on these outcomes is not known. Multicenter randomized trials or large observational studies are urgently needed to inform clinicians and patients alike.

Author Contributions: L.B., C.S. and S.B. were responsible for drafting the article, L.B. and O.B. performed the data collection, data analysis and contributed to the interpretation of the results. L.B., P.P. and G.D. participated in the conception and the design of the study. L.P. and C.S. were responsible for the critical revision of the article and approved the final version to be published. All authors have read and agreed to the published version of the manuscript.

Funding: This research received no external funding.

Conflicts of Interest: The authors declare no conflict of interest.

References

1. Guy, J.M.; Edgar, H. (1859–1942): General practitioner and radium pioneer. *J. Med. Biogr.* **2009**, *17*, 127–134. [CrossRef] [PubMed]
2. Laufer, M.R.; Sanfilippo, J.; Rose, G. Adolescent endometriosis: Diagnosis and treatment approaches. *J. Pediatr. Adolesc. Gynecol.* **2003**, *16*, S3–S11. [CrossRef]
3. Janssen, E.B.; Rijkers, A.C.M.; Hoppenbrouwers, K.; Meuleman, C.; D'Hooghe, T.M. Prevalence of endometriosis diagnosed by laparoscopy in adolescents with dysmenorrhea or chronic pelvic pain: A systematic review. *Hum. Reprod. Update* **2013**, *19*, 570–582. [CrossRef] [PubMed]
4. Dowlut-McElroy, T.; Strickland, J.L. Endometriosis in adolescents. *Curr. Opin. Obstet. Gynecol.* **2017**, *29*, 306–309. [CrossRef] [PubMed]
5. Suchońska, B.; Gajewska, M.; Zyguła, A.; Wielgoś, M. Endometriosis resembling endometrial cancer in a postmenopausal patient. *Climacteric* **2018**, *21*, 88–91. [CrossRef] [PubMed]
6. Haas, D.; Chvatal, R.; Reichert, B.; Renner, S.; Shebl, O.; Binder, H.; Wurm, P.; Oppelt, P. Endometriosis: A premenopausal disease? Age pattern in 42,079 patients with endometriosis. *Arch. Gynecol. Obstet.* **2012**, *286*, 667–670. [CrossRef]
7. Henriksen, E. Endometriosis. *Am. J. Surg.* **1955**, *90*, 331–337. [CrossRef]
8. Ranney, B.E., III. Complete operations. *Am. J. Obstet. Gynecol.* **1971**, *109*, 1137–1144. [CrossRef]
9. Nikkanen, V.; Punnonen, R. External endometriosis in 801 operated patients. *Acta Obstet. Gynecol. Scand.* **1984**, *63*, 699–701. [CrossRef]
10. Dong-Su, J.; Tae-Hee, K. Endometriosis in a Postmenopausal Woman on Hormonal Replacement Therapy. *J. Menopausal Med.* **2013**, *19*, 151–153.
11. Benjamin, M. Snyder Postmenopausal Deep Infiltrating Endometriosis of the Colon: Rare Location and Novel Medical Therapy. *Hindawi Case Rep. Gastrointest. Med.* **2018**, *2018*, 5.
12. Palep-Singh, M.; Gupta, S. Endometriosis: Associations with menopause, hormone replacement therapy and cancer. *Menopause Int.* **2009**, *15*, 169–174. [CrossRef] [PubMed]
13. Abdallah, A.A. Gastric wall endometriosis in a postmenopausal woman. *Egypt. J. Radiol. Nucl. Med.* **2016**, *47*, 1783–1786.
14. Asencio, F.; Ribeiro, H.A.; Ribeiro, P.A.; Malzoni, M.; Adamyan, L.; Ussia, A.; Gomel, V.; Martin, D.C.; Koninckx, P.R. Symptomatic endometriosis developing several years after menopause in the absence of increased circulating estrogen concentrations: A systematic review and seven case reports. *Gynecol. Surg.* **2019**, *3*, 16.
15. Streuli, I.; Gaitzsch, H.; Wenger, J.M.; Petignat, P. Endometriosis after menopause: Physiopathology and management of an uncommon condition. *Climacteric* **2017**, *20*, 138–143. [CrossRef]
16. Cumiskey, J.; Whyte, P.; Kelehan, P.; Kelehan, P.; Gibbons, D. A detailed morphologic and immunohistochemical comparison of pre- and postmenopausal endometriosis. *J. Clin. Pathol.* **2008**, *61*, 455–459. [CrossRef]
17. Kempers, R.D.; Dockerty, M.B.; Hunt, A.B.; Symmonds, R.E. Significant postmenopausal endometriosis. *Surg. Gynecol. Obstet.* **1960**, *111*, 348–356.
18. Morotti, M.; Remorgida, V.; Venturini, P.L.; Ferrero, S. Endometriosis in menopause: A single institution experience. *Arch. Gynecol. Obstet.* **2012**, *286*, 1571–1575. [CrossRef]
19. Manero, M.G.; Royo, P. Endometriosis in a postmenopausal woman without previous hormonal therapy: A case report. *J. Med. Case Rep.* **2009**, *3*, 135. [CrossRef]
20. Mehedintu, C.; Plotogea, M.N. Endometriosis still a challenge. *J. Med. Life* **2014**, *7*, 349–357.
21. Rolla, E. Writing–Review & Editing Endometriosis: Advances and controversies in classification, pathogenesis, diagnosis, and treatment. *F1000Research* **2019**, *8*. [CrossRef]

22. Saccardi, C.; Cosmi, E.; Borghero, A.; Tregnaghi, A.; Dessole, S.; Litta, P. Comparison between transvaginal sonography, saline contrast sonovaginography and magnetic resonance imaging in the diagnosis of posterior deep infiltrating endometriosis. *Ultrasound Obstet. Gynecol.* **2012**, *40*, 464–469. [CrossRef]
23. Vimercatti, A.; Achilarre, M.T.; Scardapane, A.; Lorusso, F.; Ceci, O.; Mangiatordi, G.; Angelelli, G.; Herendael, B.V.; Selvaggi, L.; Bettocchi, S. Accuracy of transvaginal sonography and contrast-enhanced magnetic resonance-colonography for the presurgical staging of deep infiltrating endometriosis. *Ultrasound Obstet. Gynecol.* **2012**, *40*, 592–603. [CrossRef] [PubMed]
24. Parveen, P.; Pinar, O.; Terry, K.L. Endometriosis: Epidemiology, Diagnosis and Clinical Management. *Curr. Obstet. Gynecol. Rep.* **2017**, *6*, 34–41.
25. Ulrich, U.; Buchweitz, O.; Greb, R.; Keckstein, J.; von Leffern, I.; Oppelt, P.; Renner, S.P.; Sillem, M.; Stummvoll, W.; De Wilde, R.L.; et al. National German Guideline (S2k): Guideline for the Diagnosis and Treatment of Endometriosis: Long Version -AWMF Registry No. 015-045. *Geburtshilfe Frauenheilkd* **2014**, *74*, 1104–1118. [PubMed]
26. Armstrong, C. ACOG updates guideline on diagnosis and treatment of endometriosis. *Am. Fam. Physician* **2011**, *1*, 83–84.
27. Kuznetsov, L.; Dworzynski, K.; Davies, M.; Overton, C. Guideline Committee. Diagnosis and management of endometriosis: Summary of NICE guidance. *BMJ* **2017**, *358*, j3935. [CrossRef]
28. Dunselman, G.A.; Vermeulen, N.; Becker, C.; Calhaz-Jorge, C.; D'Hooghe, T.; De Bie, B. ESHRE guideline: Management of women with endometriosis. *Hum. Reprod.* **2014**, *29*, 400–412. [CrossRef]
29. Schipper, E.; Nezhat, C. Video-assisted laparoscopy for the detection and diagnosis of endometriosis: Safety, reliability, and invasiveness. *Int. J. Womens Health* **2012**, *4*, 383–393.
30. Alborzi, S.; Rasekhi, A.; Shomali, Z.; Madadi, G.; Alborzi, M.; Kazemi, M.; Nohandani, A.H. Diagnostic accuracy of magnetic resonance imaging, transvaginal, and transrectal ultrasonography in deep infiltrating endometriosis. *Medicine (Baltim.)* **2018**, *97*, e9536. [CrossRef]
31. Bratila, E.; Comandașu, D.E.; Coroleucă, C.; Cîrstoiu, M.M.; Berceanu, C.; Mehedintu, C.; Bratila, P.; Vladareanu, S. Diagnosis of endometriotic lesions by sonovaginography with ultrasound gel. *Med. Ultrason* **2016**, *18*, 469–474. [CrossRef]
32. Cossi, P.; Schor, E.; Gonçalves, L.F.; Werner, H. Assessment of rectovaginal endometriosis using three-dimensional gel-infusion sonovaginography. *Ultrasound Obstet. Gynecol* **2019**, *53*, 558–560. [CrossRef]
33. Reid, S.; Lu, C.; Hardy, N.; Casikar, I.; Reid, G.; Cario, G.; Chou, D.; Almashat, D.; Condous, G. Office gel sonovaginography for the prediction of posterior deep infiltrating endometriosis: A multicenter prospective observational study. *Ultrasound Obstet. Gynecol.* **2014**, *44*, 710–718. [CrossRef] [PubMed]
34. Han, C.; Bellone, S.; Siegel, E.R.; Altwerger, G.; Menderes, G.; Bonazzoli, E.; Egkata-Takata, T.; Pettinella, F.; Bianchi, A.; Riccio, F.; et al. A novel multiple biomarker panel for the early detection of high-grade serous ovarian carcinoma. *Gynecol. Oncol.* **2018**, *149*, 585–591. [CrossRef] [PubMed]
35. Rai, N.; Champaneria, R.; Snell, K.; Mallett, S.; Bayliss, S.E.; Neal, R.D.; Balogun, M.; Kehoe, S.; Deeks, J.J.; Sundar, S.; et al. Symptoms, ultrasound imaging and biochemical markers alone or in combination for the diagnosis of ovarian cancer in women with symptoms suspicious of ovarian cancer. *Cochrane Database Syst. Rev.* **2015**, *2015*, CD011964. [CrossRef]
36. Dorien, F.O.; Fassbender, A.; Van Bree, R.; Laenen, A.; Peterse, D.P.; Vanhie, A.; Waelkens, E.; D'Hooghe, T.M. Technical Verification and Assessment of Independent Validation of Biomarker Models for Endometriosis. *Biomed. Res. Int.* **2019**, *2019*, 3673060.
37. Kennedy, S.; Bergvist, A.; Chapron, C.; D'Hooghe, T.; Dunselman, G.; Greb, R.; Hummelshoj, L.; Prentice, A. ESHRE guideline for the diagnosis and treatment of endometriosis. *Hum. Reprod.* **2005**, *20*, 2698–2704. [CrossRef]
38. Ozyurek, E.S.; Yoldemir, T.; Kalkan, U. Surgical challenges in the treatment of perimenopausal and postmenopausal endometriosis. *Climacteric* **2018**, *4*, 385–390. [CrossRef]
39. Moen, M.H.; Rees, M.; Brincat, M.; Erel, T.; Gambacciani, M.; Lambrinoudaki, I.; Schenck-Gustafsson, K.; Tremollieres, F.; Vujovic, S.; Rozenberg, S. European Menopause and Andropause Society. EMAS position statement: Managing the menopause in women with a past history of endometriosis. *Maturitas* **2010**, *67*, 94–97. [CrossRef]

40. Gemmell, L.C.; Webster, K.E.; Kirtley, S.; Vincent, K.; Zondervan, K.T.; Becker, C.M. The management of menopause in women with a history of endometriosis: A systematic review. *Hum. Reprod. Update* **2017**, *23*, 481–500. [CrossRef]
41. Oxholm, D.; Knudsen, U.B.; Kryger-Baggesen, N.; Ravn, P. Postmenopausal endometriosis. *Acta Obstet. Gynecol. Scand.* **2007**, *86*, 1158–1164. [CrossRef] [PubMed]
42. Tan, D.A.; Almaria, M.J.G. Postmenopausal endometriosis: Drawing a clearer clinical picture. *Climacteric* **2018**, *21*, 249–255. [CrossRef] [PubMed]
43. Inceboz, U. Endometriosis after menopause. *Womens Health (Lond.)* **2015**, *11*, 711–715. [CrossRef] [PubMed]
44. Somboonporn, W.; Panna, S.; Temtanakitpaisan, T.; Kaewrudee, S.; Soontrapa, S. Effects of the levonorgestrel-releasing intrauterine system plus estrogen therapy in perimenopausal and postmenopausal women: Systematic review and meta-analysis. *Menopause* **2011**, *18*, 1060–1066. [CrossRef] [PubMed]
45. Zanello, M.; Borghese, G.; Manzara, F.; Esposti, E.D.; Moro, E.; Raimondo, D.; Abdullahi, L.O.; Arena, A.; Terzano, P.; Meriggiola, M.C.; et al. Hormonal Replacement Therapy in Menopausal Women with History of Endometriosis: A Review of Literature. *Medcine* **2019**, *55*, 477. [CrossRef] [PubMed]
46. Takayama, K.; Zeitoun, K.; Gunby, R.T.; Sasano, H.; Carr, B.R.; Bulun, S.E. Treatment of severe postmenopausal endometriosis with an aromatase inhibitor. *Fertil. Steril.* **1998**, *69*, 709–713. [CrossRef]
47. Bulun, S.E.; Yang, S.; Fang, Z.; Gurates, B.; Tamura, M.; Sebastian, S. Estrogen production and metabolism in endometriosis. *Ann. N. Y. Acad. Sci.* **2002**, *955*, 75–85. [CrossRef]
48. Słopien, R.; Męczekalski, B. Aromatase inhibitors in the treatment of endometriosis. *Prz. Menopauzalny Menopause Rev.* **2016**, *15*, 43–47. [CrossRef]
49. Hajjar, L.R.; Kim, W.; Nolan, G.H.; Turner, S.; Raju, U.R. Intestinal and pelvic endometriosis presenting as a tumor and associated with tamoxifen therapy: Report of a case. *Obstet. Gynecol.* **1993**, *82* (Suppl. S2), 642–644.
50. Bardi, M.; Arnoldi, E.; Pizzocchero, G.; Pezzica, E.; Mattioni, D.; Perotti, M. Endometrioid carcinoma in pelvic endometriosis in a postmenopausal woman with tamoxifen adjuvant therapy for breast cancer: A case report. *Eur. J. Gynaecol. Oncol.* **1994**, *15*, 393–395.
51. Cohen, I.; Altaras, M.M.; Lew, S.; Tepper, R.; Beyth, Y.; Ben-Baruch, G. Ovarian endometrioid carcinoma and endometriosis developing in a postmenopausal breast cancer patient during tamoxifen therapy: A case report and review of the literature. *Gynecol. Oncol.* **1994**, *55*, 443–447. [CrossRef] [PubMed]
52. Schlesinger, C.; Silverberg, S.G. Tamoxifen-associated polyps (basalomas) arising in multiple endometriotic foci: A case report and review of the literature. *Gynecol. Oncol.* **1999**, *73*, 305–311. [CrossRef] [PubMed]
53. Okugawa, K.; Hirakawa, T.; Ogawa, S.; Kaku, T.; Nakano, H. Ovarian endometrioid adenocarcinoma arising from an endometriotic cyst in a postmenopausal woman under tamoxifen therapy for breast cancer: A case report. *Gynecol. Oncol.* **2002**, *87*, 231–234. [CrossRef] [PubMed]
54. Bese, T.; Simsek, Y.; Bese, N.; Ilvan, S.; Arvas, M. Extensive pelvic endometriosis with malignant change in tamoxifen-treated postmenopausal women. *Int. J. Gynecol. Cancer* **2003**, *13*, 376–380. [CrossRef]
55. Marie-Scemama, L.; Even, M.; De La Joliniere, J.B.; Ayoubi, J.M. Endometriosis and the menopause: Why the question merits our full attention. *Horm. Mol. Biol. Clin. Investig.* **2019**, *37*, 1. [CrossRef]
56. Brinton, L.A.; Gridley, G.; Persson, I.; Baron, J.; Bergqvist, A. Cancer risk after a hospital discharge diagnosis of endometriosis. *Am. J. Obstet. Gynecol.* **1997**, *176*, 572–579. [CrossRef]
57. Van Gorp, T.; Amant, F.; Neven, P.; Vergote, I.; Moerman, P. Endometriosis and the development of malignant tumours of the pelvis. A review of literature. *Best Pract. Res. Clin. Obstet. Gynaecol.* **2004**, *18*, 349–371. [CrossRef]
58. Somigliana, E.; Vigano, P.; Parazzini, F.; Stoppelli, S.; Giambattista, E.; Vercellini, P. Association between endometriosis and cancer: A comprehensive review and critical analysis of clinical epidemiological evidence. *Gynecol. Oncol.* **2006**, *101*, 331–341. [CrossRef]
59. Bertelsen, L.; Mellemkjær, L.; Frederiksen, K.; Kjær, S.K.; Brinton, L.A.; Sakoda, L.C.; van Valkengoed, I.; Olsen, J.H. Risk for breast cancer among women with endometriosis. *Int. J. Cancer* **2006**, *120*, 1372–1375. [CrossRef]
60. Ness, R.B. Endometriosis and ovarian cancer: Thoughts on shared pathophysiology. *Am. J. Obstet. Gynecol.* **2003**, *189*, 280–294. [CrossRef]
61. Zanetta, G.M.; Webb, M.J.; Li, H.; Keeney, G.L. Hyperestrogenism: A relevant risk factor for the development of cancer from endometriosis. *Gynecol. Oncol.* **2000**, *79*, 18–22. [CrossRef] [PubMed]

62. Mathey, M.P.; de Jolinière, J.B.; Major, A.; Pugin, F.; Monnard, E.; Fiche, M.; Sandmeier, D.; Khomsi, F.; Feki, A. Endometriotic Mass after Hysterectomy in a 61 Year Old Post-menopausal Woman: A Case Report and Update. *Front. Surg.* **2019**, *6*, 14. [CrossRef] [PubMed]
63. Charatsi, D.; Koukoura, O.; Ntavela, I.G. Gastrointestinal and Urinary Tract Endometriosis: A Review on the Commonest Locations of Extrapelvic Endometriosis. *Adv. Med.* **2018**, *2018*, 3461209. [CrossRef] [PubMed]
64. Bergqvist, A. Extragenital endometriosis: A review. *Eur. J. Surg.* **1992**, *158*, 7–12. [PubMed]
65. Popoutchi, P.; Reis Lemos, C.R.; Silva, J.C.; Nogueira, A.A.; Feres, O.; Ribeiro da Rocha, J.J. Postmenopausal intestinal obstructive endometriosis: Case report and review of the literature. *Sao Paulo Med. J.* **2008**, *126*, 190–193. [CrossRef] [PubMed]
66. Flyckt, R.; Lyden, S.; Roma, A.; Falcone, T. Post-menopausal endometriosis with inferior vena cava invasion requiring surgical management. *Hum. Reprod.* **2011**, *26*, 2709–2712. [CrossRef] [PubMed]
67. Milone, M.; Mollo, A.; Musella, M.; Maietta, P.; Fernandez, L.M.S.; Shatalova, O.; Conforti, A.; Barone, G.; De Placide, G.; Milone, F. Role of colonoscopy in the diagnostic work-up of bowel endometriosis. *World J. Gastroenterol.* **2015**, *21*, 4997–5001. [CrossRef]
68. Thomsen, L.H.; Schnack, T.H.; Buchardi, K.; Hummelshoj, L.; Missmer, S.A.; Forman, A.; Blaakaer, J. Risk factors of epithelial ovarian carcinomas among women with endometriosis: A systematic review. *Acta Obstet. Gynecol. Scand.* **2017**, *96*, 761–778. [CrossRef]
69. Jones, K.D.; Owen, E.; Berresford, A.; Sutton, C. Endometrial adenocarcinoma arising from endometriosis of the rectosigmoid colon. *Gynecol. Oncol.* **2002**, *86*, 220–222. [CrossRef]
70. Ponticelli, C.; Graziani, G.; Montanari, E. Ureteral Endometriosis: A Rare and Underdiagnosed Cause of Kidney Dysfunction. *Nephron Clin. Pract.* **2010**, *114*, c89–c94. [CrossRef]
71. Stewart, W.W.; Ireland, G.W. Vesical endometriosis in a postmenopausal woman: A case report. *J. Urol.* **1977**, *118*, 480–481. [CrossRef]
72. Habuchi, T.; Okagaki, T.; Miyakawa, M. Endometriosis of Bladder after Menopause. *J. Urol.* **1991**, *145*, 361–363. [CrossRef]

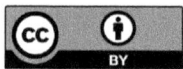

© 2020 by the authors. Licensee MDPI, Basel, Switzerland. This article is an open access article distributed under the terms and conditions of the Creative Commons Attribution (CC BY) license (http://creativecommons.org/licenses/by/4.0/).

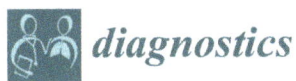

Article

Does Endometriosis Influence the Embryo Quality and/or Development? Insights from a Large Retrospective Matched Cohort Study

Ana M. Sanchez [1], Luca Pagliardini [1,*], Greta C. Cermisoni [2], Laura Privitera [2], Sofia Makieva [1], Alessandra Alteri [2], Laura Corti [2], Elisa Rabellotti [2], Massimo Candiani [2] and Paola Viganò [1]

1. Reproductive Sciences Laboratory, Division of Genetics and Cell Biology, IRCCS San Raffaele Scientific Institute, 20132 Milano, Italy; asg.alcala@gmail.com (A.M.S.); makieva.sofia@hsr.it (S.M.); vigano.paola@hsr.it (P.V.)
2. IRCCS San Raffaele Scientific Institute, Obstetrics and Gynecology Unit, 20132 Milano, Italy; cermisoni.greta@hsr.it (G.C.C.); privitera.laura@hsr.it (L.P.); alteri.alessandra@hsr.it (A.A.); corti.laura@hsr.it (L.C.); rabellotti.elisa@hsr.it (E.R.); candiani.massimo@hsr.it (M.C.)
* Correspondence: pagliardini.luca@hsr.it

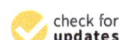

Received: 31 December 2019; Accepted: 31 January 2020; Published: 3 February 2020

Abstract: In vitro fertilization can be an effective tool to manage the endometriosis-associated infertility, which accounts for 10% of the strategy indications. Nevertheless, a negative effect of endometriosis on IVF outcomes has been suggested. The aim of this study was to evaluate the potential effect of endometriosis in the development of embryos at cleavege stage in assisted reproduction treatment cycles. A total of 429 cycles from women previously operated for moderate/severe endometriosis were compared with 851 cycles from non-affected women. Patients were matched by age, number of oocyte retrieved and study period. A total of 3818 embryos in cleavage stage have been analyzed retrospectively. Overall, no difference was found between women with and without endometriosis regarding the number of cleavage stage embryos obtained as well as the percentage of good/fair quality embryos. Excluding cycles in which no transfers were performed or where embryos were frozen in day three, no difference was observed for blastulation rate or the percentage of good/fair blastocysts obtained. Despite similar fertilization rate and number/quality of embryos, a reduction in ongoing pregnancy rate was observed in patients affected, possibly due to an altered endometrial receptivity or to the limited value of the conventional morphological evaluation of the embryo.

Keywords: embryo quality; endometriosis; blastulation rate; ongoing pregnancy

1. Introduction

Endometriosis affects from 10% to 15% of reproductive aged women and around 30% of women suffering from infertility, which is up to 10-fold more frequent than in the general population (0.5–5%) [1,2]. Mechanisms that have been postulated to explain the low fecundity of women with endometriosis include altered folliculogenesis, reduced quality and cytoplasmic mitochondrial content of oocytes, oocyte/embryo exposure to a hostile inflammatory environment (macrophages, cytokines and vasoactive substances in the peritoneal fluid), anatomical dysfunctions of the tubes and/or ovary and reduced endometrial receptivity [3].

Assisted Reproduction Technology (ART) can be an effective tool to manage the endometriosis-associated infertility, which indeed accounts for 10% of the strategy indications. Nevertheless, a negative effect of endometriosis on ART outcomes has been suggested [4–6], albeit not consistently [7–9]. Both oocyte/embryo number and quality have been claimed to be affected by the disease [3]. Lower implantation rates have been as well postulated. However, the reasons to explain the suboptimal performance of ART in endometriosis patients are still poorly understood and can only be hypothesized.

Data from meta-analyses are only partially informative in this regard. The meta-analysis from Barnhart et al. [4] including data from 22 studies, found a reduction in fertilization and implantation rates in women with endometriosis when compared with non-affected women or with women that underwent ART for tubal-factor infertility only [4]. Harb and colleagues, including 27 studies, reported a reduction in clinical pregnancy rate in women with stage III/IV endometriosis compared to controls, but not a reduction in live births [10]. No differences in reproductive outcomes were found by Barbosa and colleagues between women with and without endometriosis. Only the number of oocytes at the time of retrieval was found to be lower in women affected [11].

Unfortunately, few studies have considered the consequence of endometriosis on the embryological outcomes. This aspect is important considering that in recent years the reproductive medicine laboratories are trying to optimize embryo transfer strategies, e.g., by transferring the embryo later in development instead of transfer at an early stage. Additionally, single blastocyst transfer has been preferred to a simultaneous transfer of multiple early stage embryos.

In association with the importance of the embryonic developmental stage for an optimal uterine transfer, it is critical to elucidate factors that can threaten embryonic competence to progress in a healthy pregnancy. In this context, Freis and colleagues have recently reported that the relative morphokinetic profiles of embryos from patients with endometriosis are altered, indicating a negative impact of the disease independently from the stage on the embryo quality [12]. Herein, we have scrutinized the plausible negative impact of endometriosis on embryonic parameters in a retrospective non-interventional analysis of ART cycles in our center.

The aim of the study was to investigate whether endometriosis affects embryo development and/or quality. The primary outcome of the study was the quality of cleavage stage (day 3) embryo in terms of number of cells, cell fragmentation and symmetry. Secondary outcome measures were (1) fertilization rate, (2) number of good/fair embryos at cleavage stage, (3) blastulation rate (defined as percentage of total blastocyst obtained per number of fertilized eggs, excluding cycles in which embryos were transferred or frozen in day 3, (4) good/fair blastocyst formation rate, and (5) ongoing pregnancy rate (defined when the pregnancy had completed ≥ 20 weeks of gestation per transfer).

2. Results

The baseline characteristics of the cycles for the two study groups are presented in Table 1: the maternal age, Body Mass Index (BMI), antral follicle count and Anti-Müllerian hormone (AMH) levels were significantly different between the two groups.

Table 1. Basal characteristics of the analyzed cycles.

Parameters	Controls $n = 851$	Endometriosis $n = 429$	p-Value
Age (years)	37.5 ± 3.6	36.9 ± 3.6	0.003
BMI (kg/m^2)	22.4 ± 3.6	21.6 ± 2.9	0.004
Antral follicle count	8.0 ± 4.7	6.3 ± 3.2	<0.001
AMH (ng/mL)	1.9 ± 2.5	1.5 ± 1.9	<0.001
Total dose FSH administered (IU)	3112 ± 1600	3419 ± 1641	0.003
E2 at the time of hCG administration (pg/mL)	1635 ± 1084	1562 ± 1057	0.18
Number of oocytes retrieved	5.8 ± 4.4	5.9 ± 4.6	0.90
Number of oocytes retrieved/1000 IU of FSH	2.8 ± 4.1	2.2 ± 2.6	0.09
Percentage of mature oocytes	75 (50–100)	71 (50–100)	0.25
Sperm Count (×10^6/mL)	31.2 ± 28.2	37.5 ± 26.9	<0.001
% Motility (a + b)	35 (20–50)	40 (30–50)	<0.001

Data are presented as mean ± standard deviation or median (interquartile range). IU: International Units; BMI: Body Mass Index; AMH: Anti-Müllerian Hormone; FSH: Follicle-Stimulating Hormone; hCG: Human Chorionic Gonadotropin.

Age was used as a variable to match cases and controls and a significant difference was observed between the two groups, that was however limited as an absolute value and for which the subsequent results were adjusted. The semen characteristics of the endometriosis and non-endometriosis groups are shown in Table 1. Sperm concentration and motility were significantly different between the groups. No differences were found in the levels of estrogen at the time of hCG administration and in the number of oocytes retrieved per 1000U of FSH (2.8 ± 4.1 controls vs 2.2 ± 2.6 endometriosis patients, $p = 0.09$).

The number of oocytes retrieved in both groups was similar (5.8 ± 4.4 non-endometriosis vs 5.8 ± 4.6 endometriosis patients, $p = 0.9$). We did not find any statistically significant differences in the percentage of MII oocytes (75% (50–100%) controls vs. 71% (50–100%) endometriosis patients, $p = 0.25$) and in fertilization rate (75% (50–100%) controls vs. 75% (50–100%) endometriosis patients, adjusted $p = 0.85$) (Table 2).

Table 2. ART outcomes in the two studied groups.

Header Parameters	Controls $n = 851$	Endometriosis $n = 429$	Estimated Difference	95% CI Lower Limit	95% CI Upper Limit	p-Value	corrected p-Value *
Fertilization rate, median (IQR)	75 (50–100)	75 (50–100)	0.0	−4.5	4.5	0.29	0.85
Cleavage rate, median (IQR)	100 (100–100)	100 (100–100)	0.0	0.0	0.0	0.33	0.83
Cleavage stage embryos (n), mean ± SD	3.5 ± 2.6	3.7 ± 2.6	0.1	−0.2	0.5	0.42	0.77
Number of cells of the embryos, mean ± SD	7.0 ± 1.4	6.9 ± 1.5	−0.1	−0.3	0.1	0.22	0.42
Percentage of good/fair embryos, median (IQR)	56 (25–100)	50 (17–88)	−5.6	−15.0	4.0	0.20	0.36
Blastulation rate, median (IQR)	50 (25–67)	50 (25–67)	0.0	−6.0	6.0	0.68	0.22
Percentage of good/fair blastocysts, median (IQR)	50 (33–80)	50 (25–75)	0.0	−7.0	7.0	0.43	0.88

Data are presented as mean ± standard deviation or median (IQR: interquartile range). * Adjusted for age, BMI, semen parameters and percentage of mature oocytes.

Overall, we did not find any difference regarding the number of cleavage stage embryos obtained (3.5 ± 2.6 non-endometriosis vs. 3.7 ± 2.6 endometriosis patients, adjusted $p = 0.77$) and the mean number of blastomers of the embryos (7.0 ± 1.4 controls vs 6.9 ± 1.5 endometriosis patients, adjusted $p = 0.42$) between endometriosis women and controls. In addition, the percentage of good/fair quality embryos was similar (56% (25–100%) controls vs. 50% (17–88%) endometriosis patients, adjusted $p = 0.36$). Excluding cycles whereby embryos were transferred or frozen in day 3, no difference was found in blastulation rate between the two groups (50% (25–67%) controls vs. 50% (25–67%) endometriosis patients, adjusted $p = 0.22$). Finally, we calculated the percentage of good/fair blastocysts obtained and we did not find any difference (50% (33–80%) controls vs. 50% (25–75%) endometriosis patients, adjusted $p = 0.88$) (Table 2). No differences in terms of the number of cancelled cycles and/or freeze-all cycles were found between both groups (Supplementary Table S1).

Despite similar fertilization rate and number/quality of embryos obtained, we found a reduction in ongoing pregnancy after adjusting for the number of transferred embryos and the day of transfer (cleavage or blastocyst stage) (24.2% in controls vs. 17.8% in endometriosis group, adjusted OR = 0.62; 95% CI 0.40–0.94, $p = 0.02$) (Table 3).

A similar reduction was observed when considering transfers at day 3 or day 5, separately. Similar results were observed in terms on ongoing pregnancy rate considering frozen embryo transfers (Supplementary Table S2).

Table 3. Embryo transfer details and ongoing pregnancy rate.

Header Parameters	Controls $n = 516$	Endometriosis $n = 253$	p-Value
Number of transferred embryos, mean ± SD	1.6 ± 0.7	1.7 ± 0.7	0.10
Day 3 transfers	1.7 ± 0.7	1.8 ± 0.7	0.16
Day 5 transfers	1.3 ± 0.5	1.4 ± 0.5	0.20
Number of transfers (%)			
Day 3 transfers	396 (76.7)	192 (75.9)	0.86
Day 5 transfers	120 (23.3)	61 (24.1)	
Ongoing pregnancy rate (95% CI)			
All transfers	24.2 (20.7–28.1)	17.8 (13.5–22.9)	0.05
Day 3 transfers	21.7 (17.9–26.0)	15.1 (10.7–20.9)	0.07
Day 5 transfers	32.5 (24.8–41.3)	26.2 (16.8–38.4)	0.49
Adjusted Odds Ratios for ongoing pregnancy rate, (95% CI)			
All transfers *	-	0.62 (0.40–0.94)	0.02
Day 3 transfers **	-	0.58 (0.35–0.97)	0.04
Day 5 transfers **	-	0.76 (0.35–1.64)	0.49

* Adjusted for age, BMI, semen parameters, percentage of mature oocytes, day of the transfer and number of transferred embryos. ** Adjusted for age, BMI, semen parameters, percentage of mature oocytes and number of transferred embryos.

3. Discussion

This is, at least to the best of our knowledge, the largest study that analyzed the potentially deleterious effect of endometriosis on the in vitro development of embryos in ART cycles. We were unable to demonstrate an impact of endometriosis on day three embryo quality and developmental potential. The fertilization rates and percentage of good/fair quality embryos from endometriosis patients and controls were also similar. Moreover, in patients who did not perform a fresh transfer and/or freeze embryos at day three, we did not find any statistical difference in blastulation rate and/or the percentage of good/fair quality blastocyst obtained. Therefore, in the light of the results obtained, women with endometriosis may as well opt for the blastocyst culture in the presence of good quality embryo at day three in order to improve the reproductive outcomes after ART [13].

A limited number of studies have been published in relation to the in vitro development of embryos obtained from women with endometriosis. Coccia and colleagues published one of the first studies in 2011. In contrast to our results, the total number of embryos obtained in their ART cycles was significantly different between the endometriosis and the control group represented by women with tubal factor infertility. This discrepancy may be explained by methodological differences: firstly, they did not match for age, number of oocytes retrieved and/or study period. Secondly, only 3 oocytes were used for conventional IVF (under Italian law 40/2004 for ART) [5]. Finally, in endometriosis patients they notably observed a decrease in the number of oocytes retrieved, which could have impacted the number of embryos obtained. The reduction in the number of oocytes retrieved demonstrated in several studies may be ascribed to the detrimental effect of previous surgical treatments rather than to the disease itself. It is for this reason that we have decided to match our population for this parameter in order to avoid this bias. More recently, two studies have been performed using the time-lapse technology for the assessment of embryo morphokinetics in endometriosis patients [12,14]. In the study by Demirel and colleagues, the endometriosis population was constituted only by patients with a diagnosis of endometrioma. Specifically, the authors compared embryos derived from oocytes collected from an ovary affected by an endometrioma to embryos developed from oocytes from the contralateral healthy ovary failing to find differences in terms of morphokinetic parameters [14]. In contrast, Freis and colleagues compared embryo morphokinetics between women with and without endometriosis (tubal factor) showing a poorer relative kinetics in embryos from affected patients [12].

The group of Song and colleagues have demonstrated that the number of mature follicles and good embryos, and fertilization and blastulation rates were reduced in women with endometriosis compared with women with a male factor indication [15]. In line with our results, Benaglia and colleagues found that, in women with bilateral endometriomas, despite the lower number of oocytes retrieved, no differences could be observed in terms of fertilization rate, number of embryos obtained and rate of top-quality embryos per oocyte used compared to controls without the disease [16]. Finally, in a recent work of Muteshi and colleagues they demonstrated that endometriosis may affect embryo development due to a reduction in the percentage of women with endometriosis that reach blastocyst transfer compare with women with unexplain infertility [17]. Therefore, overall, data from the literature addressing the embryological parameters in ART cycles of women with endometriosis are very controversial.

Unfortunately, some of these previous studies are characterized by important limitations: firstly, the small sample size resulting in lack of statistical power and secondly, the lack of matching for age or number of collected oocytes or of corrections for confounders. These limitations of others have been addressed in the present study and represent the main strength of our work. Based on our results, at present, there are no strong evidence to set up a different culture or transfer strategy or to change the conventional embryological practice in ART cycles performed in patients with endometriosis.

In terms of IVF clinical outcomes, despite a similar number of transferred embryos and no differences in the day of transfer between women with and without the disease, we found a reduction in the ongoing pregnancy rates in the affected women. Several meta-analyses describing the effect of endometriosis on IVF outcomes have been published, again with contradictory results [4,6,10,11]. The inclusion of studies with very heterogeneous populations both for endometriosis and control group represents the main problem of these meta-analyses. The presence of side causes of infertility other than endometriosis are also rarely considered in the meta-analyses [18]. It should be considered that our endometriosis population consists of all operated women for a stage III/IV disease and that we have corrected for confounders potentially affecting fertility such as BMI and sperm motility/concentration.

In terms of ongoing pregnancy rate we found a similarly reduction of ongoing pregnancy rate in the endometriosis group compared to the control one in the freeze all cycles, consequently we cannot conclude that endometriosis women have better ART outcome after freeze all cycle. This data is supported by the recent study of Roque and colleagues [19], that reported that even if initial studies showed that the freeze-all strategy could be beneficial for certain groups of infertility including endometriosis patients [20], there is still lack of evidence to support its routine use not only for indications as endometriosis but also for implantation failure. In conclusion the data published until now is very controversial about better ART outcomes after freeze all cycles in endometriosis patients [19].

Two hypotheses can be put forward to explain our overall findings. The first is that, given the lack of differences in terms of embryo development/quality and blastulation rate in the endometriosis group, one might wonder whether an altered endometrial receptivity may explain the reduced chance of an ongoing pregnancy in affected women. Inflammatory-related changes in gene expression and/or a progesterone resistance in the endometrium of women with endometriosis might have a role [21,22]. This again represents a critical point. Some endometrial receptivity defects have been detected in these women [23]. However, data from clinical IVF egg donation program do not support this idea [24].

The second explanation is that the conventional morphological evaluation of the embryos, even at day 3 of development, may scarcely predict the embryo competence in these patients. Embryo grade has some value in predicting implantation [25] but, certainly, the embryo selection based on morphologic criteria could be imprecise [26] and may be even more imprecise in women with endometriosis. Indeed, oocytes have been demonstrated to more likely fail in vitro maturation and to have lower cytoplasmic mitochondrial content in women affected compared to women with other causes of infertility [3]. The time-lapse technology might be of value in this context.

The main limitation of our study is its retrospective design; however, for the calculation of the main outcome, no clinical decision/intervention has been done between the time of fertilization and day three of culture. The majority of the women from control group did not undergo laparoscopy prior to ART, therefore we cannot totally exclude the possibility that we incorrectly selected some affected women. This possibility could have influenced the study power to detect differences between the two groups. Similarly to the study of Barbosa and colleges, we have considered to include in the control group all the other women (without the diagnosis of endometriosis), because applying any other selection criterion would be arbitrary and might introduce biases [11]. Finally, the heterogeneity of the control group in terms of cause of infertility represents another bias that should be considered. Indeed, the different prevalence of causes underlying infertility could significantly impact on the quality of the embryos analyzed. This problem may be one of the reasons for the disagreements in terms of ART outcomes in the different studies already published and might have impacted the outcomes related to the blastulation rate and pregnancies. Similarly, although all cases were post-surgical, parameters such as moderate/severe disease, the different intervals from surgical management of endometriosis and ART treatment may have affected the results. In fact, based on a recent study of AlKudmani and collaborators [27], significant higher IVF ongoing pregnancy rates were observed in women with endometriosis after 6–25 months from the surgery compared with women with endometriosis undergoing IVF after 25 months from surgery [27]. In addition, another limitation of the study is the lack of information about the location of endometriosis lesions (superficial endometriosis, deep infiltrating endometriosis, endometriomas). At this regard, in a recent study of Ashrafi and colleagues [28], they demonstrated that the presence of deep infiltration endometriosis in the presence or not of endometrioma was associated with an 80% decrease in the probability of live births in comparison with that of a control group, but no information concerning the performance in the laboratory has been published.

In conclusion, we report that endometriosis does not compromise fertilization rate, the quality of cleavage stage embryos, of the blastocysts and blastulation rates. Thus, this study does not support the need to tailor embryo transfer strategy to the incidence of endometriosis. On the other hand, we found a reduction in ongoing pregnancy in patients affected, but an explanation for this observation warrants certainty. These results can help in understanding the mechanisms by which endometriosis impacts fertility.

4. Materials and Methods

4.1. Patients

This is a single center retrospective study matched cohort study, non-interventional, including patients who underwent ART cycles at the San Raffaele Hospital (Milan, Italy) from 2013 to 2017.

We performed a matched cohort study of the variables believed to be confounding (in order to avoid confounding) in our study design and to ensure an equal distribution among affected and non-affected.

Endometriosis was laparoscopically diagnosed in all the patients before ART treatment and classified according to the American Society for Reproductive Medicine ASRM criteria into stage III-IV (moderate/severe) [29], all women received a complete surgical treatment for endometriosis and all the lesions were removed. A total of 309 women were included in the study with a total of 429 ART cycles performed.

The control group were patients without a laparoscopic diagnosis or a history of endometriosis and did not have any ultrasonographic evidence of endometriotic ovarian cyst at the time of the cycle, including patients with tubal factor (female infertility caused by diseases, obstructions, damage, scarring, congenital malformations or other factors that impede the descent of a fertilized or unfertilized ovum into the uterus through the Fallopian tubes), male factor (patients that underwent at least two consecutive semen analyses, both showing below-standard values for normal semen parameters according to the World Health Organization (WHO) criteria), poor ovarian reserve (Bologna criteria definition [30]), idiopatic or patients that underwent PGT-M cycles for monogenic diseases (diseases that not affect the fertility of the couple, excluding genetic causes of male infertility) (Supplementary Table S3). Controls were matched to cases on a ratio 2:1 by age (± 1 year), number of oocytes retrieved (± 1 oocyte) and study period (± 4 months). A total of 851 cycles from control women were included in the analysis (from 766 patients). A total of 3818 cleavage stage embryos (day 3) have been analyzed.

Data collection followed the principles defined in the Declaration of Helsinki; all women undergoing ART in San Raffaele Hospital routinely provide informed consent for their clinical data and anonymized records to be used for research purposes in general. Women who denied this consent were excluded. Local Institutional Review Board approval (ID: BC-GINEOS, date of approval: 09/02/2012, San Raffaele Hospital Ethics Committee) for the use of clinical data for research studies was obtained.

4.2. Controlled Ovarian Stimulation, In Vitro Fertilization, Embryo Culture and Grading

All patients were treated with a GnRH antagonist protocol as previously descrived [31]. Oocyte collection was performed 36 h after triggering of ovulation. In both groups, in order to avoid biases in the evaluation of the number of MII oocytes and in the fertilization rate, only ICSI cycles were considered for analysis (that represents the 91% of the study group before matching). ICSI cycles were performed as previously descrived [32]. Sixteen-eighteen hours after ICSI, oocytes were checked for fertilization and transfer to 10% of Serum substitute supplement (SSS, Irvine, CA, USA)-supplemented Cleavage medium (REF ART-1026, Sage In-Vitro Fertilization, inc. Trumbull, CT, USA) under oil. Embryos were checked at 68 ± 1 after ICSI, and an embryo evaluation was performed according to the Istanbul consensus [33]. Briefly, the embryo quality was calculated in terms of number of blastomers, cell fragmentation and symmetry. A good/fair-quality embryo was considered that with ≥7 cells on day 3, with a fragmentation rate lower than 10% and a stage-specific cell size for majority of cells [33].

For evaluation of blastocyst data [cultured into 10% of Serum substitute supplement (SSS, Irvine, CA, USA)-supplemented Blastocyst medium (REF ART-1029, Sage In-Vitro Fertilization, inc. Trumbull, CT, USA)], only patients who did not perform transfer or freezing of day 3 embryos were included, hence patients who underwent prolonged culture of the whole cohort of embryos formed.

Blastocyst evaluation was performed according to the Istanbul Consensus (116 ± 2 h post insemination) [33] as previously described [31]. Based on the rating, a good/fair blastocyst was defined as expanded or hatched blastocyst with both an inner cell mass and multicellular trophectoderm scored good or fair or at least one of them scored as good or fair. Blastocysts were never frozen before the expanded stage.

All embryo transfers were scheduled in day 3 (at cleavage stage). The decision to transfer in day 3 or delay the embryo culture to day 5 (blastocyst stage) depends on the evaluation of the quality and the number of cleave stage embryos at day 3 and woman's age. Criteria for blastocyst culture were the presence at day 3 of 4 or more embryos and at least 2 good/fair embryos in women younger than 38 years old and three good/fair embryos for women aged 38 years and older [34].

In our laboratory, an embryo quality control is performed with a biannual frequency, together with other subjective evaluations (i.e., oocyte quality control, preimplantation diagnosis biopsy control) among the embryologists as previously described [31,35]. In any case, for this specific study, we choose to enroll in the study only cycles in which the quality of the embryos was evaluated every day by the same embryologist (P.V.) who is assigned to this specific task most of the time. To prove the reliability of the evaluations, we have measured the ability of conventional morphological analysis of the embryo to predict ART outcomes. An odds ratio of 5.7 (95% confidence interval 1.7–19.5, $p = 0.006$) for ongoing pregnancy was found after a single embryo transfer of day 3 good/fair embryos compared to poor quality embryos.

4.3. Statistical Methods

All continuous variables are presented as mean ± standard deviation (SD) or median with interquartile range (IQR). Normality of variables distributions were checked using the Kolmogorov–Smirnoff test. Student's *t*-test, Mann–Whitney U test and chi-squared test were used as appropriate. Multivariate analysis was conducted using the generalized estimating equation (GEE) approach, thus making it possible to use multiple cycles of the same patient and at the same time allow the analysis of variables with non-normal distribution. Age, BMI, concentration and motility of sperm and percentage of mature oocytes were used as predictors in the GEE model in order to obtain adjusted estimation for the differences between cases and controls. The ongoing pregnancy rate was adjusted for day of transfer and also for the number of transferred embryos and the adjusted estimate was reported as odds ratio (OR) with 95% confidence interval (95% CI). Differences were considered statistically significant if $p < 0.05$. Data were analyzed using the SPSS software 17.0 (SPSS, Inc., Chicago, IL, USA).

Supplementary Materials: The following are available online at http://www.mdpi.com/2075-4418/10/2/83/s1.

Author Contributions: Conceptualization, A.M.S., L.P. and G.C.C.; methodology, A.M.S., L.P., G.C.C. and L.C.; data curation, A.M.S., G.C.C., L.P., A.A, L.C. and E.R.; statistical analysis, A.M.S. and L.P.; writing—original draft preparation, A.M.S., L.P., S.M. and P.V.; writing—review and editing, A.M.S., L.P., G.C.C., L.P., S.M., A.A., L.C., E.R., M.C. and P.V. All authors have read and agreed to the published version of the manuscript.

Funding: This research received no external funding.

Conflicts of Interest: The authors declare no conflict of interest.

Abbreviations

ART	Assisted Reproduction Technology
BMI	Body Mass Index
AMH	Anti-Müllerian Hormone
IU	International Unit
FSH	Follicle-Stimulating Hormone
IQR	Interquantile Range
SD	Standard Deviation
IVF	In Vitro Fertilization
GnRH	Gonadotropin-Releasing Hormone
hCG	human Chorionic Gonadotropin
PGT-M	Preimplantation Genetic Testing for Monogenic/single gene diseases.

References

1. Somigliana, E.; Vigano, P.; Benaglia, L.; Busnelli, A.; Berlanda, N.; Vercellini, P. Management of Endometriosis in the Infertile Patient. *Semin. Reprod. Med.* **2017**, *35*, 31–37. [PubMed]
2. Zondervan, K.T.; Becker, C.M.; Koga, K.; Missmer, S.A.; Taylor, R.N.; Viganò, P. Endometriosis. *Nat. Rev. Dis. Primers.* **2018**, *4*, 9. [CrossRef] [PubMed]
3. Sanchez, A.M.; Vanni, V.S.; Bartiromo, L.; Papaleo, E.; Zilberberg, E.; Candiani, M.; Orvieto, R.; Viganò, P. Is the oocyte quality affected by endometriosis? A review of the literature. *J. Ovarian Res.* **2017**, *10*, 43. [CrossRef] [PubMed]
4. Barnhart, K.; Dunsmoor-Su, R.; Coutifaris, C. Effect of endometriosis on in vitro fertilization. *Fertil. Steril.* **2002**, *77*, 1148–1155. [CrossRef]
5. Coccia, M.E.; Rizzello, F.; Mariani, G.; Bulletti, C.; Palagiano, A.; Scarselli, G. Impact of endometriosis on in vitro fertilization and embryo transfer cycles in young women: A stage-dependent interference. *Acta Obs. Gynecol. Scand.* **2011**, *90*, 1232–1238. [CrossRef]
6. Hamdan, M.; Omar, S.Z.; Dunselman, G.; Cheong, Y. Influence of endometriosis on assisted reproductive technology outcomes: A systematic review and meta-analysis. *Obs. Gynecol.* **2015**, *125*, 79–88. [CrossRef]

7. Bukulmez, O.; Yarali, H.; Gurgan, T. The presence and extent of endometriosis do not effect clinical pregnancy and implantation rates in patients undergoing intracytoplasmic sperm injection. *Eur. J. Obs. Gynecol. Reprod. Biol.* **2001**, *96*, 102–107. [CrossRef]
8. Al-Fadhli, R.; Kelly, S.M.; Tulandi, T.; Lin Tan, S. Effects of different stages of endometriosis on the outcome of in vitro fertilization. *J. Obs. Gynaecol. Can.* **2006**, *28*, 888–891. [CrossRef]
9. Opøien, H.K.; Fedorcsak, P.; Byholm, T.; Tanbo, T. Complete surgical removal of minimal and mild endometriosis improves outcome of subsequent IVF/ICSI treatment. *Reprod. Biomed. Online.* **2011**, *23*, 389–395. [CrossRef]
10. Harb, H.M.; Gallos, I.D.; Chu, J.; Harb, M.; Coomarasamy, A. The effect of endometriosis on in vitro fertilisation outcome: A systematic review and meta-analysis. *BJOG* **2013**, *120*, 1308–1320. [CrossRef]
11. Barbosa, M.A.; Teixeira, D.M.; Navarro, P.A.; Ferriani, R.A.; Nastri, C.O.; Martins, W.P. Impact of endometriosis and its staging on assisted reproduction outcome: Systematic review and meta-analysis. *Ultrasound Obs. Gynecol.* **2014**, *44*, 261–278. [CrossRef] [PubMed]
12. Freis, A.; Dietrich, J.E.; Binder, M.; Holschbach, V.; Strowitzki, T.; Germeyer, A. Relative Morphokinetics Assessed by Time-Lapse Imaging Are Altered in Embryos From Patients With Endometriosis. *Reprod. Sci.* **2018**, *25*, 1279–1285. [CrossRef] [PubMed]
13. Glujovsky, D.; Farquhar, C.; Quinteiro Retamar, A.M.; Alvarez Sedo, C.R.; Blake, D. Cleavage stage versus blastocyst stage embryo transfer in assisted reproductive technology. *Cochrane Database Syst. Rev.* **2016**, *6*, CD002118. [CrossRef] [PubMed]
14. Demirel, C.; Bastu, E.; Aydogdu, S.; Donmez, E.; Benli, H.; Tuysuz, G.; Keskin, G.; Buyru, F. The Presence of Endometrioma Does Not Impair Time-Lapse Morphokinetic Parameters and Quality of Embryos: A Study On Sibling Oocytes. *Reprod. Sci.* **2016**, *23*, 1053–1057. [CrossRef]
15. Song, Y.; Liu, J.; Qiu, Z.; Chen, D.; Luo C1 Liu, X.; Hua, R.; Zhu, X.; Lin, Y.; Li, L.; Liu, W.; et al. Advanced oxidation protein products from the follicular microenvironment and their role in infertile women with endometriosis. *Exp. Med.* **2018**, *15*, 479–486. [CrossRef]
16. Benaglia, L.; Bermejo, A.; Somigliana, E.; Faulisi, S.; Ragni, G.; Fedele, L.; Garcia-Velasco, J.A. In vitro fertilization outcome in women with unoperated bilateral endometriomas. *Fertil. Steril.* **2013**, *99*, 1714–1719. [CrossRef]
17. Muteshi, C.M.; Ohuma, E.O.; Child, T.; Becker, C.M. The effect of endometriosis on live birth rate and other reproductive outcomes in ART cycles: A cohort study. *Hum. Reprod. Open.* **2018**, *2018*, hoy016. [CrossRef]
18. Senapati, S.; Sammel, M.D.; Morse, C.; Barnhart, K.T. Impact of endometriosis on in vitro fertilization outcomes: An evaluation of the Society for Assisted Reproductive Technologies Database. *Fertil. Steril.* **2016**, *106*, 164–171. [CrossRef]
19. Roque, M.; Nuto Nóbrega, B.; Valle, M.; Sampaio, M.; Geber, S.; Haahr, T.; Humaidan, P.; Esteves, S.C. Freeze-all strategy in IVF/ICSI cycles: An update on clinical utility. *Panminerva Med.* **2019**, *61*, 52–57. [CrossRef]
20. Bourdon, M.; Santulli, P.; Maignien, C.; Gayet, V.; Pocate-Cheriet, K.; Marcellin, L.; Chapron, C. The deferred embryo transfer strategy improves cumulative pregnancy rates in endometriosis-related infertility: A retrospective matched cohort study. *PLoS ONE.* **2018**, *13*, e0194800. [CrossRef]
21. Patel, B.G.; Rudnicki, M.; Yu, J.; Shu, Y.; Taylor, R.N. Progesterone resistance in endometriosis: Origins, consequences and interventions. *Acta. Obs. Gynecol. Scand.* **2017**, *96*, 623–632. [CrossRef]
22. Makieva, S.; Giacomini, E.; Ottolina, J.; Sanchez, A.M.; Papaleo, E.; Viganò, P. Inside the endometrial cell signaling subway: Mind the gap(s). *Int. J. Mol. Sci.* **2018**, *21*, 19. [CrossRef] [PubMed]
23. Lessey, B.A.; Kim, J.J. Endometrial receptivity in the eutopic endometrium of women with endometriosis: It is affected, and let me show you why. *Fertil. Steril.* **2017**, *108*, 19–27. [CrossRef] [PubMed]
24. Miravet-Valenciano, J.; Ruiz-Alonso, M.; Gómez, E.; Garcia-Velasco, J.A. Endometrial receptivity in eutopic endometrium in patients with endometriosis: It is not affected, and let me show you why. *Fertil. Steril.* **2017**, *108*, 28–31. [CrossRef] [PubMed]
25. Weitzman, V.N.; Schnee-Riesz, J.; Benadiva, C.; Nulsen, J.; Siano, L.; Maier, D. Predictive value of embryo grading for embryos with known outcomes. *Fertil. Steril.* **2010**, *93*, 658–662. [CrossRef] [PubMed]
26. Ebner, T.; Moser, M.; Sommergruber, M.; Tews, G. Selection based on morphological assessment of oocytes and embryos at different stages of preimplantation development: A review. *Hum. Reprod. Update.* **2003**, *9*, 251–262. [CrossRef]

27. AlKudmani, B.; Gat, I.; Buell, D.; Salman, J.; Zohni, K.; Librach, C.; Sharma, P. In Vitro Fertilization Success Rates after Surgically Treated Endometriosis and Effect of Time Interval between Surgery and In Vitro Fertilization. *J Minim Invasive Gynecol.* **2018**, *25*, 99–104. [CrossRef]
28. Ashrafi, M.; Arabipoor, A.; Hemat, M.; Salman-Yazdi, R. The impact of the localisation of endometriosis lesions on ovarian reserve and assisted reproduction techniques outcomes. *J. Obs. Gynaecol.* **2019**, *39*, 91–97. [CrossRef]
29. American Society for Reproductive Medicine—ASRM. Revised American Society for Reproductive Medicine classification of endometriosis. *Fertil. Steril.* **1996**, *67*, 817–882. [CrossRef]
30. Ferraretti, A.P.; La Marca, A.; Fauser, B.C.; Tarlatzis, B.; Nargund, G.; Gianaroli, L.; ESHRE working group on Poor Ovarian Response Definition. ESHRE consensus on the definition of 'poor response' to ovarian stimulation for in vitro fertilization: The Bologna criteria. *Hum. Reprod.* **2011**, *26*, 1616–1624. [CrossRef]
31. Vanni, V.S.; Somigliana, E.; Reschini, M.; Pagliardini, L.; Marotta, E.; Faulisi, S.; Paffoni, A.; Vigano', P.; Vegetti, W.; Candiani, M.; et al. Top quality blastocyst formation rates in relation to progesterone levels on the day of oocyte maturation in GnRH antagonist IVF/ICSI cycles. *PLoS ONE.* **2017**, *12*, e0176482. [CrossRef] [PubMed]
32. Rubino, P.; Viganò, P.; Luddi, A.; Piomboni, P. The ICSI procedure from past to future: A systematic review of the more controversial aspects. *Hum. Reprod. Update.* **2016**, *22*, 194–227. [CrossRef] [PubMed]
33. ALPHA Scientists In Reproductive Medicine; ESHRE Special Interest Group Embryology. Istanbul consensus workshop on embryo assessment: Proceedings of an expert meeting. *Reprod. Biomed. Online.* **2011**, *22*, 632–646. [CrossRef] [PubMed]
34. Cutting, R.; Morroll, D.; Roberts, S.A.; Pickering, S.; Rutherford, A.; BFS; ACE. Elective single embryo transfer: Guidelines for practice British Fertility Society and Association of Clinical Embryologists. *Hum. Fertil.* **2008**, *11*, 131–146. [CrossRef] [PubMed]
35. Gentilini, D.; Somigliana, E.; Pagliardini, L.; Rabellotti, E.; Garagnani, P.; Bernardinelli, L.; Papaleo, E.; Candiani, M.; Di Blasio, A.M.; Viganò, P. Multifactorial analysis of the stochastic epigenetic variability in cord blood confirmed an impact of common behavioral and environmental factors but not of in vitro conception. *Clin. Epigenetics.* **2018**, *10*, 77. [CrossRef] [PubMed]

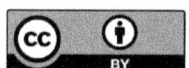

© 2020 by the authors. Licensee MDPI, Basel, Switzerland. This article is an open access article distributed under the terms and conditions of the Creative Commons Attribution (CC BY) license (http://creativecommons.org/licenses/by/4.0/).

MDPI
St. Alban-Anlage 66
4052 Basel
Switzerland
Tel. +41 61 683 77 34
Fax +41 61 302 89 18
www.mdpi.com

Diagnostics Editorial Office
E-mail: diagnostics@mdpi.com
www.mdpi.com/journal/diagnostics

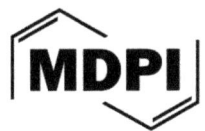